# WALKING ----→

## NEW ORLEANS

**Walking New Orleans: 33 Historic Neighborhoods, Waterfront Districts, and Recreational Wonderlands**

Copyright © 2015 and 2021 by Barri Bronston

Cover design: Scott McGrew
Interior design: Lora Westberg
Cover photo: © Inge Johnsson/Alamy Stock Photo
Interior photos: © by Barri Bronston, except where noted on page
Cartography: Steve Jones
Indexing: Rich Carlson

**Library of Congress Cataloging-in-Publication Data**

Names: Bronston, Barri, 1958– author.
Title: Walking New Orleans : 33 historic neighborhoods, waterfront districts, and
    recreational wonderlands / Barri Bronston.
Other titles: 33 historic neighborhoods, waterfront districts, and recreational wonderlands
Description: Second edition. | Birmingham, AL : Wilderness Press, [2021]
Identifiers: LCCN 2020056694 (print) | LCCN 2020056695 (ebook) |
    ISBN 9781643590356 (paperback) | ISBN 9781643590363 (ebook)
Subjects: LCSH: New Orleans (La.)—Guidebooks. | New Orleans (La.)—Tours. |
    Walking—Louisiana—New Orleans—Guidebooks.
Classification: LCC F379.N53 B76 2021 (print) | LCC F379.N53 (ebook) | DDC 917.63/3504—dc23
LC record available at https://lccn.loc.gov/2020056694
LC ebook record available at https://lccn.loc.gov/2020056695

Published by ⚘ **WILDERNESS PRESS**
An imprint of AdventureKEEN
2204 First Ave. S., Ste. 102
Birmingham, AL 35233
800-678-7006, fax 877-374-9016

Visit wildernesspress.com for a complete list of our books and for ordering information. Contact us at our website, at facebook.com/wildernesspress1967, or at twitter.com/wilderness1967 with questions or comments. To find out more about who we are and what we're doing, visit blog.wildernesspress.com.

Distributed by Publishers Group West
Manufactured in the United States of America

**SAFETY NOTICE** Although Wilderness Press and the author have made every attempt to ensure that the information in this book is accurate at press time, they are not responsible for any loss, damage, injury, or inconvenience that may occur to anyone while using this book. You are responsible for your own safety and health while following the walking trips described here. Always check local conditions, know your own limitations, and consult a map.

For the latest information about destinations in this book that have been affected by the coronavirus, please check the "Points of Interest" listings following the walks. For updates about the coronavirus in New Orleans and Louisiana, see ready.nola.gov/incident/coronavirus and ldh.la.gov/coronavirus.

# WALKING ------→
# NEW ORLEANS

33 Historic Neighborhoods, Waterfront Districts,
and Recreational Wonderlands

2nd Edition

Barri Bronston

 **WILDERNESS PRESS** ... *on the trail since 1967*

# Acknowledgments

Writing this book was a challenging endeavor that I could not have fulfilled without the help of many individuals and organizations.

First of all, I would like to thank Wilderness Press for recognizing the importance of New Orleans as a walking city and former acquisitions editor Susan Haynes for giving me this amazing opportunity. I would also like to thank Molly Merkle, chief operating officer, for giving me the green light to write a second edition five years later. In addition, I'd like to thank managing editor Holly Cross, along with the production team of cartographer Steve Jones, typesetter Annie Long, proofreader Rebecca Henderson, and indexer Rich Carlson for putting all the pieces together and adding the finishing touches.

I also want to thank my sister Donna Goldenberg for her wonderful photography, along with her husband, Eric, and son, Trevor, who accompanied Donna and me on a walk through the breathtaking Jean Lafitte Barataria Preserve. Thanks to Janet Pesses, DeeGee Liniado, and Laura Fuhrman for joining me on some of the walks. And thank you to my good friend Kathy Anderson, of Kathy Anderson Photography, for my beautiful new portrait.

Thanks go out to Kathryn Hobgood Ray for her help with the Algiers Point neighborhood, to Beth Donze for her expertise on Faubourg St. John, and to Lisanne Brown for steering me to Crescent Park and other funky spots in Bywater. A big thank-you to Eddie Bronston, my former husband but still good friend, for lending his musical expertise for the walk covering Faubourg Marigny and Frenchmen Street. I'd also like to acknowledge Mike Strecker, my boss at Tulane University, for reviewing the University section and making sure that I included some of Tulane's most important landmarks.

For the Lafitte Greenway and Jean Lafitte Barataria Preserve walks, I relied on their materials and maps, and for those I would like to thank both of them. I also want to thank the New Orleans Tourism Marketing Corporation and the St. Tammany Parish Tourist & Convention Commission for providing me with some terrific images.

Although she no longer lives in New Orleans—but knows it almost as well as I do—my daughter and best friend, Sally Bronston, served as a great sounding board as I pondered various aspects of the book, especially what bars and restaurants to include. Thanks, Sally! You may live in Washington, D.C., but NOLA will always be home.

—*Barri Bronston*

# Author's Note

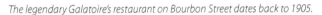

I was born in New Orleans in the late 1950s, and except for four years attending college in Missouri and another year living in Arkansas, I've spent pretty much my entire life in what is often referred to as one of the world's most fascinating cities.

For most of that time, I was a journalist, an experience that gave me an up-close encounter with the people and places that have made New Orleans one of the coolest, craziest, and most captivating destinations on the map.

Still, as a native, I tended to take my city for granted. Not until I took on this book in the summer of 2013 did I really start to get it—that "it" being the heap of honors that have been bestowed on New Orleans in recent years, among them being named one of the world's top 10 cities by *Travel & Leisure,* a best American city for foodies by *Condé Nast Traveler,* and one of six trips that will change your life by *Coastal Living.* When I was tasked with writing this second edition in the summer of 2019, it came as no surprise to see even more accolades—the South's Best Food City (*Southern Living,* March 2020); 25 Best Places to Visit in 2020 (*Forbes,* 2019); and Most Excellent City Overall (TripAdvisor, 2019).

New Orleans has certainly overcome more than its fair share of challenges—and continues to do so—but I'm prouder than ever to be a native and resident of New Orleans.

*The legendary Galatoire's restaurant on Bourbon Street dates back to 1905.*

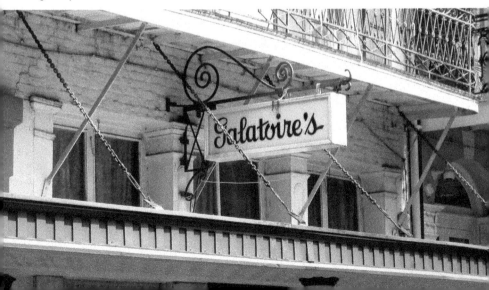

# Table of Contents

# Walking New Orleans

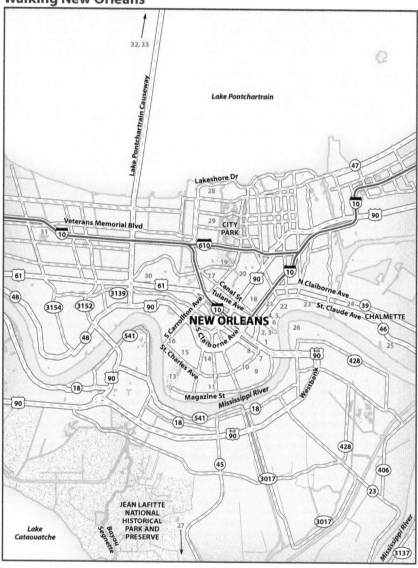

Numbers on this locator map correspond to walk numbers.

# Introduction

When the first edition of *Walking New Orleans* came out in the spring of 2015, New Orleanians were just a few months away from commemorating the 10-year anniversary of Hurricane Katrina. The powerful, life-altering storm was one of our country's most horrific disasters, destroying approximately 80 percent of New Orleans, killing more than 1,800 people, and forcing hundreds of thousands to flee the city, some forever. Even worse, it had some politicians arguing against spending federal dollars to rebuild a city that lies 7 feet below sea level.

Fortunately, their whining fell on deaf ears, and New Orleans was transformed back into one of the most captivating, culturally diverse, and entertaining cities in the world. Public education improved, the movie business boomed, and the culinary and music scenes flourished.

From the moment the book came out, I began keeping notes for what I hoped would be a second edition down the road. Just as I expected, the notes took up one page after another. Among the Crescent City's newest attractions were the Lafitte Greenway, a 2.6-mile linear park connecting Mid-City with the French Quarter; several food halls, including one in the Warehouse District and another on St. Claude Avenue; and JAMNOLA, a whimsical exhibition space in Bywater. The Louisiana Children's Museum moved into its bigger and better digs at City Park, and the culinary scene continued to flourish, with the addition of such restaurants as Justine, Saba, Meril, and Gris Gris. We also saw an influx of new museums, among them The Sazerac House, the Museum of the Southern Jewish Experience, and the Petite Jazz Museum.

I began discussing the possibility of a second edition with Molly Merkle at Adventure-KEEN in July 2019, and we both agreed that the timing was right for a new *Walking New Orleans*. As I embarked on the research, it was clear that most of the walks would have to be revised in some fashion. For example, I remapped the Faubourg Marigny chapter to include Hotel Peter and Paul, an award-winning church transformation and home of the wildly popular bar and café The Elysian. I extended the Lakeview walk to include New Basin Canal Park, a linear greenspace between West End Boulevard and Pontchartrain Boulevard. And I changed up the Bywater walk to include the super cool JAMNOLA, a celebration of art and music. I also added four new walks: Old Metairie, St. Claude Avenue, the Lafitte Greenway, and Madisonville.

Things took a bit of a challenging—and depressing—turn in March 2020 when the COVID-19 pandemic shut down most of the city: bars, restaurants, museums, theaters, shops, and more. As the health crisis continued into the summer, it was apparent that some of these places would not survive. It saddened me to have to remove some of these from the original book—the Audubon Nature Institute Insectarium (some exhibits have moved to the Aquarium of the Americas); K-Paul's Louisiana Kitchen, the legendary Cajun restaurant made famous by the late chef Paul Prudhomme; Bootsy's Funrock'n, a vintage variety shop on Magazine Street; and Chiba, a popular sushi spot on Oak Street. As of this writing, dozens of restaurants and bars remained temporarily closed. But it didn't make sense to label them as such since most are hoping to reopen by the spring of 2021.

Even with all of the uncertainty, there thankfully has been no ban on walking. In fact, the pandemic has made leisurely outdoor strolls more popular than ever. So grab some comfy shoes and take to the streets of New Orleans. There isn't a better way to see and appreciate the city than by foot, be it through the historic Irish Channel, the funky Marigny, the colorful Bywater, or any of the other 30 walks in this book.

As you would on any walking tour, in any city, use common sense: Walk in groups, and avoid walking after dark. And as you're trekking away, be on the lookout for broken sidewalks and potholes, which sadly are common sights in many New Orleans neighborhoods.

Oh, and don't forget your water—especially if you plan to conquer one of these walks during the city's infamous sweltering summer.

*Opposite: Bourbon Street at twilight*
*photo by Shutterstock/Sean Pavone*

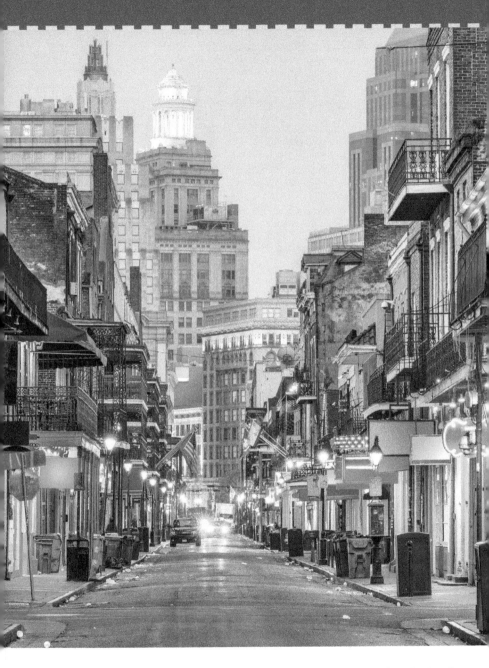

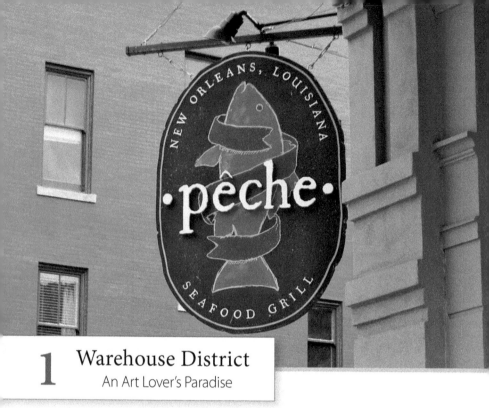

# 1 Warehouse District
## An Art Lover's Paradise

*Above: Pêche Seafood Grill, known for its vast selection of coastal seafood, is an essential stop for any foodie traveling to New Orleans.   photo by Donna Goldenberg*

BOUNDARIES: St. Charles Ave., Poydras St., Convention Center Blvd., Andrew Higgins Dr.
DISTANCE: 1.8 miles
PARKING: Lots, garages, metered parking
PUBLIC TRANSIT: St. Charles Ave. Streetcar

The Warehouse District, also called the Arts District, is by far one of the coolest neighborhoods in New Orleans, its establishment an answer to the urban blight that replaced a once-thriving industrial area. The Contemporary Arts Center pioneered the effort in 1976, converting a dilapidated building into a showcase for visual and performing artists.

Over the next quarter of a century, the area experienced a complete transformation, and today it is home to some of the city's preeminent museums, galleries, restaurants, and clubs. Countless buildings have been converted into luxury condo developments, making the Warehouse District one of the most desirable neighborhoods in town.

Museums include the National World War II Museum, the Ogden Museum of Southern Art, the Confederate Memorial Hall Museum, and the Museum of the Southern Jewish Experience. Julia Street boasts some of the city's top art galleries, among them the Arthur Roger Gallery, Gallery 600 Julia, and Jonathan Ferrara Gallery.

The culinary scene is equally vibrant. Eateries range from upscale Emeril's and Tommy's to the trendy and hip Auction House food hall and Pêche Seafood Grill. For drinks—and fun—gathering spots include NOSH Wine Lounge, Flamingo's A-Go-Go, Barcadia, Lucy's Retired Surfer Bar, and Manning's, the sports bar and restaurant owned by Archie Manning, former New Orleans Saints quarterback and father of former NFL quarterbacks Eli and Peyton.

# Walk Description

Begin your walk at the corner of Howard Avenue and Carondolet Street in front of the wine store ❶ Kiefe and Co., which offers a wide variety of wines, spirits, and specialty foods. Directly across Howard Avenue is the ❷ Museum of the Southern Jewish Experience, which through exhibits, collections, and programs focuses on the history of Southern Jews and encourages understanding of and appreciation for identity, diversity, and acceptance. Continue walking down Howard past the ❸ New Orleans Culinary and Hospitality Institute, also known as NOCHI, which in addition to training aspiring chefs features classes for home cooking enthusiasts, a café, and private event space.

Walk to the intersection of St. Charles Avenue and Andrew Higgins Boulevard to the ❹ former location of Lee Circle, known for its bronze statue of General Robert E. Lee, commander of the Confederate Army during the Civil War. Lee was also a slaveholder, and for many New Orleans residents, his statue was a symbol of racism and white supremacy. In the aftermath of the Charleston church shooting, the Lee statue and three other Confederate monuments were removed. Renaming considerations were underway as of this writing.

Walk a block down Andrew Higgins across Camp Street, and turn left. To the right is the ❺ Contemporary Arts Center, known for its bold, sometimes daring displays of visual and performing arts. To the left is the ❻ Confederate Memorial Hall Museum, which houses artifacts from the Civil War, including the personal belongings of soldiers along with weapons, flags, and uniforms.

Adjacent to the Confederate Museum is the ❼ Ogden Museum of Southern Art, which showcases the visual arts of the American South, including the works of Clementine Hunter, George Dureau, and Ida Kohlmeyer. The museum, named after Southern art collector and philanthropist Roger Ogden, offers live music every Thursday night, film screenings related to Ogden's collections, and an impressive array of educational programming.

Continue walking down Camp to Julia Street. At the corner of Camp and Julia is one of the many art galleries that populate the Warehouse District, ⑧ Gallery 600 Julia. Housed in an 1832 building listed on the National Register of Historic Places, the gallery showcases the works of Louisiana artists, both new and established.

Cross Julia and continue walking down Camp. On the left is the ⑨ Martine Chaisson Gallery, which, like so many of the galleries in the Warehouse District, represents both emerging and established contemporary artists. Toward the end of the block, to the right, is the ⑩ Old St. Patrick's Church, which is also on the National Register of Historic Places. The church celebrated its first Mass in 1840. At the time, services took place in a small wooden structure. Longing to worship in the same splendor that the French citizenry did at nearby St. Louis Cathedral, the Irish community rallied support for its own house of worship, and the Gothic-style Old St. Patrick's was born.

Two blocks past St. Patrick's is the ⑪ John Minor Wisdom US Court of Appeals Building, headquarters of the Fifth Circuit Court of Appeals, which hears cases from Louisiana, Texas, and Mississippi. Built in 1915 in the Italian Renaissance Revival style, the three-story marble-and-granite building features a cornice inscribed with the names of former chief justices of the US Supreme Court. The building is named for John Minor Wisdom, who served on the appellate court from 1957 until his death in 1999. Wisdom was a highly respected judge who promoted civil rights through landmark decisions involving school desegregation and voter rights.

Directly across from the courthouse is ⑫ Lafayette Square, the second-oldest park in New Orleans. From March to June, the park is home to the weekly "Wednesdays in the Square," a concert series sponsored by the Young Leadership Council. It is also a gathering spot for LUNA Fête (Light Up New Orleans Arts), an annual holiday celebrating the arts community through light, art, and technology.

Look across the square and you'll see ⑬ Gallier Hall, one of New Orleans's most iconic landmarks. Dedicated in 1853, the Greek Revival structure served as City Hall for a century and continues today as a special-events venue and occasional set location for movies and TV shows, including *NCIS: New Orleans*. On Mardi Gras Day, the mayor of New Orleans toasts the kings of the Zulu and Rex parades here.

Turn right on Lafayette Street and walk seven blocks to Convention Center Boulevard. This stretch will take you behind the Hale Boggs Federal Building and Courthouse to Fulton Street, a block-long entertainment mall featuring an array of restaurants and bars. Every winter, Harrah's New Orleans presents "Miracle on Fulton Street," converting the walkway into a wonderland of lights, decorations, and snowfall. Among the restaurants on Fulton is ⑭ Manning's, an upscale sports bar owned by former New Orleans Saints quarterback Archie Manning in partnership with

Harrah's. The restaurant features 30 flat-screen TVs, a sports anchor desk, and memorabilia from Louisiana's first family of football—Archie and sons Peyton and Eli—and various Louisiana teams. A row of comfy recliners faces the bar's megascreen.

At Convention Center Boulevard, turn right and walk three blocks to Julia Street. Across the boulevard is the ⓮ **Outlet Collection at Riverwalk**, a high-end outlet mall, and the Ernest N. Morial Convention Center, named after the first black mayor of New Orleans. At 1.1 million square feet, the center is the sixth largest in the United States.

Turn right on Julia at ⓰ **Mulate's**, a popular Cajun restaurant where you can try such Louisiana fare as fried alligator and stuffed catfish, as well as test your Cajun two-step skills on the dance floor.

From Mulate's, walk six blocks down Julia to Magazine Street. This stretch features some of the city's most iconic restaurants, including ⓱ **Emeril's New Orleans**, the flagship restaurant of celebrity chef Emeril Lagasse, at the corner of Tchoupitoulas Street. Other restaurants along Julia or in the general vicinity are Meril, Lagasse's casual restaurant, and Compere Lapin, whose chef and owner is *Top Chef: New Orleans* runner-up Nina Compton.

Among the art galleries on Julia are ⓲ **LeMieux Galleries**, ⓳ **Søren Christensen**, ⓴ **Jonathan Ferrara Gallery**, and ㉑ **Arthur Roger Gallery**. All invite visitors to stop in and browse. Julia Street is the center of two of the most popular arts events in town—White Linen Night and Art for Arts' Sake. The galleries also present art walks on the first Saturday night of every month.

Turn left on Magazine Street. To the left is ㉒ **Pêche Seafood Grill**, a James Beard Award–winning restaurant, which, since opening to rave reviews in 2013, continues to be one of the city's most popular dining spots. Across the street is ㉓ **Auction House Market**, a food hall boasting an array of cuisines from Indian to Filipino. On that same block is ㉔ **Flamingo A-Go-Go**, billed as the "go-to spot for outdoor day drinking, group gaming, bottomless brunching, and puppy play dates."

Walk two blocks to Andrew Higgins Boulevard, home of the ㉕ **National World War II Museum** (see sidebar on page 8). Through interactive exhibits, oral histories, and vignettes, the museum tells the story of the so-called War That Changed the World. The museum's Stage Door Canteen presents war-era entertainment from big-band favorites to the Victory Belles singing group (think the Andrews Sisters). Stop by the ㉖ **Higgins Hotel**, named after Andrew Higgins, who designed and built more than 20,000 boats in New Orleans that were used in World War II. The hotel features an Art Deco ambience, a French restaurant called Café Normandie, and Rosie's on the Roof, a rooftop bar.

Turn right at Andrew Higgins and head two blocks to the circle and back to the starting point at Howard and Carondolet.

# National World War II Museum

When the National World War II Museum opened as the National D-Day Museum in 2000, there were just under 6 million surviving veterans of the so-called War That Changed the World. As of 2020, the number had dwindled to just over 325,000.

According to the U.S. Department of Veterans Affairs, veterans are dying at a rate of 296 a day, making the museum's mission—to ensure that all generations understand the price of freedom and be inspired by what they learn—that much more crucial.

Named by travel website TripAdvisor in 2018 as the third best museum in the United States and the eighth best in the world, the National World War II Museum is fulfilling its mission through extraordinary exhibits that explain why the war was fought, how it was won, and what it means today.

The museum campus consists of six buildings, each dedicated to a central theme that gives visitors an opportunity to experience the war through the eyes of those who lived it. Exhibits include uniforms, weaponry, vehicles, medals, diaries, letters, artwork, photographs, and other mementos, along with oral histories and personal vignettes. The Solomon Victory Theater is home to the exclusive Tom Hanks production *Beyond All Boundaries*, a 4-D film that explains the war through dazzling special effects, archival footage, and first-person accounts. The "Road to Berlin" exhibit is a 32,000-square-foot multimedia experience that recounts the drama and personal sacrifices surrounding America's fight to defeat the Axis powers and preserve freedom.

Entertainment abounds as well, from Rat Pack and Elvis Presley tribute shows to performances by the Victory Belles, a 1940s-style singing group. If you plan to make a day of it, grab lunch at The American Sector or the Jeri Nims Soda Shop. Or head to neighboring Café Normandie at the Higgins Hotel.

## Points of Interest

1. Keife and Co.  keifeandco.com, 801 Howard Ave., 504-523-7272
2. Museum of the Southern Jewish Experience  msje.org, 818 Howard Ave., 504-345-8585
3. New Orleans Culinary and Hospitality Institute  nochi.org, 1519 Carondolet St., 504-525-2433
4. The former Lee Circle  St. Charles Avenue at Lee Circle
5. Contemporary Arts Center  cacno.org, 900 Camp St., 504-528-3805
6. Confederate Memorial Hall Museum  confederatemuseum.com, 922 Camp St., 504-523-4522
7. Ogden Museum of Southern Art  ogdenmuseum.org, 925 Camp St., 504-539-9650
8. Gallery 600 Julia  gallery600julia.com, 600 Julia St., 504-895-7375
9. Martine Chaisson Gallery  martinechaissongallery.com, 727 Camp St., 504-302-7942
10. Old St. Patrick's Church  oldstpatricks.org, 724 Camp St., 504-525-4413
11. John Minor Wisdom US Court of Appeals Building  uscourts.gov, 600 Camp St., 504-310-7700

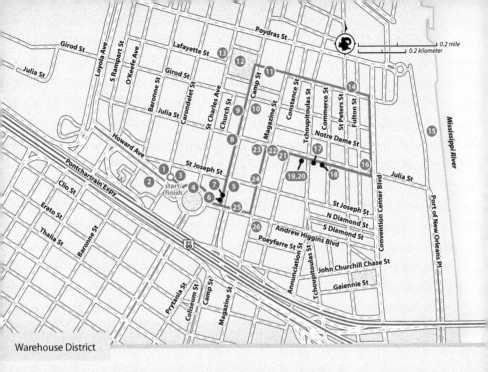

**Warehouse District**

12 Lafayette Square nola.gov/parks-and-parkways/parks-squares/lafayette-square, bounded by St. Charles Ave., Camp St., N. Maestri St., and S. Maestri St.; 504-658-3200

13 Gallier Hall nola.gov/gallier-hall, 545 St. Charles Ave., 504-658-3627

14 Manning's caesars.com/harrahs-new-orleans/restaurants/mannings-sports-bar-and-grill, 519 Fulton St., 504-593-8118

15 Outlet Collection at Riverwalk riverwalkneworleans.com, 500 Port of New Orleans, 504-522-1555

16 Mulate's mulates.com, 201 Julia St., 504-522-1492

17 Emeril's New Orleans emerilsrestaurants.com, 800 Tchoupitoulas St., 504-528-9393

18 LeMieux Galleries lemieuxgalleries.com, 332 Julia St., 504-522-5988

19 Søren Christensen sorengallery.com, 400 Julia St., 504-569-9501

20 Jonathan Ferrara Gallery jonathanferraragallery.com, 400-A Julia St., 504-522-5471

21 Arthur Roger Gallery arthurrogergallery.com, 432 Julia St., 504-522-1999

22 Pêche Seafood Grill pecherestaurant.com, 800 Magazine St., 504-522-1744

23 Auction House Market auctionhousemarket.com, 801 Magazine St., 504-372-4321

24 Flamingo A-Go-Go flamingonola.com, 869 Magazine St., 504-577-2202

25 National World War II Museum nationalww2museum.org, 945 Magazine St., 504-527-6012

26 Higgins Hotel higginshotelnola.com, 1000 Magazine St., 504-528-1941

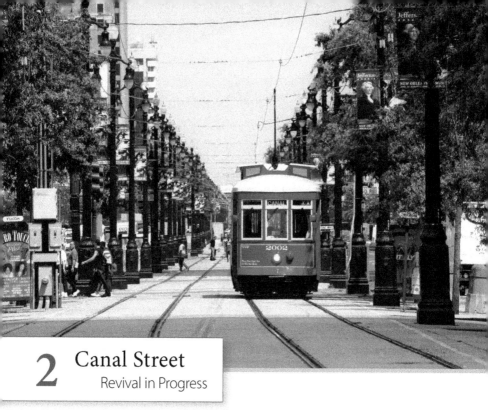

# 2 Canal Street
## Revival in Progress

*Above: Canal Street, once the city's premier shopping destination, is making a steady comeback, thanks to the efforts of the nonprofit Canal Street Redevelopment Corporation.*
photo courtesy of New Orleans Tourism Marketing Corp.

BOUNDARIES: Canal St., Basin St., Convention Center Blvd.
DISTANCE: 1.93 miles
PARKING: Lots, garages, metered parking
PUBLIC TRANSIT: St. Charles Ave. Streetcar

Ask older natives of New Orleans about their memories of Canal Street, and you'll likely see their eyes light up as they recall dressing up in their finest attire and heading downtown to what was once the city's equivalent of Fifth Avenue. Back in the day, Canal Street—named for a canal that was never built—was the city's primary shopping destination, home to such classic department stores as Gus Mayer, Godchaux's, Kreeger's, Holmes, Krauss, and Maison Blanche.

As enclosed shopping malls began sprouting up in the suburbs and many of these stores began opening multiple locations, Canal—which separates the French Quarter from the Central

Business District—took a major hit. Crowds began to thin, opting for the convenience of the malls, near which New Orleanians were moving in droves. By the late 1990s, only a couple of specialty stores, Adler's and Rubenstein Bros., remained.

To be sure, Canal Street was not the same—not that it had turned into a ghost town, but the quality of the shopping had been reduced to fast-food restaurants and discount stores peddling electronics, souvenirs, and T-shirts. Today, many of those outlets still exist, but a major revitalization effort has made Canal Street a destination once again, with upscale stores, luxury hotels and apartments, theaters, and restaurants now in the mix.

# Walk Description

Begin at 333 Canal Street, home of ❶ the Shops at Canal Place and the Westin Hotel New Orleans. Stores at Canal Place include Saks Fifth Avenue, Brooks Brothers, Tiffany and Co., Vineyard Vines, Tory Burch, and Louis Vuitton.

Walk one block. Between North Peters and Decatur Streets is the historic ❷ U.S. Custom House, a mammoth granite building erected over 33 years in the 19th century. Designated as a National Historic Landmark, the building housed the Audubon Butterfly Garden and Insectarium until 2020, when it became a casualty of the COVID-19 pandemic. The good news is that Audubon Institute relocated some of the Insectarium exhibits to the nearby Audubon Aquarium of the Americas.

Continue down Canal Street just past Chartres Street, where you'll see the ❸ Palace Café, a Brennan family restaurant known for such contemporary Creole dishes as crabmeat cheesecake, duck-and-roasted-garlic gumbo, and white-chocolate bread pudding. The restaurant is housed in another historic structure: the old Werlein's Building, which until 1990 was one of *the* places in New Orleans to buy sheet music, pianos, and other musical instruments.

As you continue walking down Canal Street, you'll pass several luxury hotels, including the ❹ Ritz-Carlton, where jazz favorite Jeremy Davenport performs regularly in the Davenport Lounge. The Ritz is housed in what was once the headquarters of Maison Blanche, one of the city's most popular department stores. Similarly, the Hyatt French Quarter is located in the old D. H. Holmes building. Holmes, another of New Orleans's legendary department stores, was known as much for its exterior clock as it was for its merchandise. If you were meeting friends downtown, you likely were meeting them "under the clock at D. H. Holmes"—a location immortalized in *A Confederacy of Dunces,* the beloved comic novel by John Kennedy Toole.

Walk two blocks and cross North Rampart Street. To the right is the venerable ❺ Saenger Theatre, home to the Broadway in New Orleans series. Listed on the National Register of Historic

Places, the Saenger opened in 1927 as a venue for silent movies and stage shows. The theater's trademark feature was its European-style interior, designed by architect Emile Weil to resemble an Italian Baroque courtyard. As part of the design, Weil installed dozens of tiny lights in the ceiling, arranging them as constellations of the night sky. The design made the Saenger the South's grandest theater and the city's preeminent place to experience "moving pictures." In 2005, the Saenger was destroyed by Hurricane Katrina, the storm's floodwaters and winds causing millions of dollars in damage. The Broadway series moved to the nearby Mahalia Jackson Theatre for the Performing Arts, where it remained until September 2013 when the Saenger unveiled its magnificent renovated digs. Costing an estimated $53 million, the restoration combines the grandness of the past with state-of-the-art performance features such as an updated orchestra pit, a deeper stage, and first-class sound and lighting systems. The rebirth of the Saenger was considered a major step in the revitalization of Canal Street.

One block past the Saenger, on your right as you approach the intersection of Canal and Basin Streets, note the statue of Venezuelan military and political giant Simón Bolívar, who led the fight for Latin American independence from Spain in the 1800s. The 12-foot-high cast-granite statue is one of three monuments to Central and South American heroes that make up the Garden of the Americas, which honors the ties between New Orleans and Latin America. The other statues are of Mexican statesman Benito Juárez (Basin and Conti), who lived in Faubourg Marigny (see Walk 22) during the 1840s, and Francisco Morazán (Basin and St. Louis), who served as president of the Federal Republic of Central America—which comprised present-day Costa Rica, El Salvador, Guatemala, Honduras, and Nicaragua—from 1830 to 1839.

Just past the monument, at 1201 Canal, is yet another former retail outlet: the site of Krauss Company, once the largest department store in the South. Now a luxury condominium development, Krauss closed in 1997, leaving behind a legacy of faithful shoppers who relished the store's old-fashioned ways of doing business. In addition to being the first store in the city to install air-conditioning and escalators (known as mechanical stairways), Krauss boasted such departments as notions, fabrics, and foundations, along with a lunch counter that served New Orleans cuisine.

Cross Canal at Basin Street. The center of Canal—which like all medians in New Orleans is called the neutral ground—is where streetcars pass, so be extra-cautious as you walk to the other side of the street. At Canal and Basin is the ❻ Joy Theater, another of the city's longtime entertainment venues. Opened in 1947 as a movie house, it was one of four movie theaters (along with the Orpheum, State Palace, and Saenger) that populated downtown. Faced with growing competition from multitheater complexes with stadium seating, the Joy shut down in

2003. It remained closed until 2011, when it reopened as a state-of-the-art venue for live music, theatrical performances, and other special events.

From the Joy, continue walking down Canal Street toward the river. Walk three blocks to Roosevelt Way. The 121-year-old ⑦ Roosevelt Hotel, just off Canal Street, is well worth a side visit, especially during December, when its grand block-long lobby is converted to a winter wonderland complete with thousands of twinkling lights, a New Orleans–themed gingerbread village, and a white-birch canopy. In addition, the hotel is home to the famed Sazerac Bar and the acclaimed Italian eatery Domenica. Like so many of the city's historic buildings, the luxury hotel sustained extensive damage from Hurricane Katrina, and restoring it cost nearly $150 million. When it reopened as part of the Waldorf Astoria hotel group, it won rave reviews from critics and guests alike.

As you continue down Canal, you'll notice numerous chain stores, many of which occupy the spaces that once housed some of the city's premier department stores. Sports Plus, at 828 Canal, is housed in the old Godchaux's building. CVS, at 800 Canal, was once Gus Mayer. In the middle of the block, at 824 Canal, is the home of the Boston Club, probably the city's most exclusive men's social club. Many of its members belong to blue-blood Carnival groups such as Rex and Comus. Until 1992, Rex, King of Carnival, toasted the Queen of Carnival at reviewing stands erected outside the Boston Club on Mardi Gras Day. That royal tradition now takes place outside the nearby Hotel InterContinental.

At 772 Canal Street is ⑧ Adler's, the city's oldest jewelry store. Adler's opened in 1898 in the French Quarter but outgrew that location and eventually moved to Canal. Even when their retail neighbors were closing up shop, Adler's never gave up on Canal. Neither did nearby Rubenstein Bros., an upscale men's clothing store that opened at the corner of Canal and St. Charles in 1924 and continues to thrive today as ⑨ Rubensteins.

Continue walking down Canal Street past Rubensteins and various other shops and hotels. At the corner of Canal and Magazine Street is ⑩ the Sazerac House, a three-story cocktail museum dedicated to the history and customs of the Sazerac and other New Orleans libations. Featuring a fully functional distillery, the museum offers complimentary self-guided tours and tastings along with drink recipes for you to take home. The walk ends at ⑪ Harrah's New Orleans, at the corner of Canal and Convention Center Boulevard. As of this writing, the hotel-casino was planning a major rebranding under the name Caesars New Orleans. The $352-million renovation will include a hotel, new dining options, and other amenities.

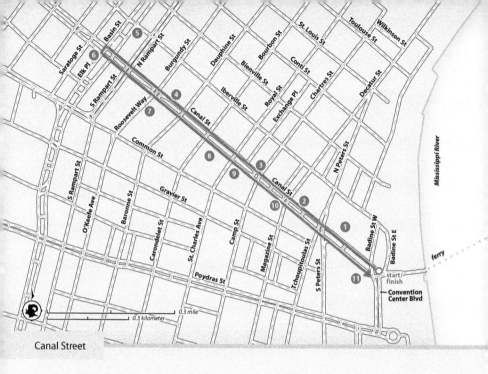

## Points of Interest

1. The Shops at Canal Place  canalplacestyle.com, 333 Canal St., 504-522-9200

2. U.S. Custom House  423 Canal St., 504-670-2391

3. Palace Café  palacecafe.com, 605 Canal St., 504-523-1661

4. Ritz-Carlton  ritzcarlton.com/en/hotels/new-orleans, 921 Canal St., 504-524-1331

5. Saenger Theatre  saengernola.com, 1111 Canal St., 504-525-1052

6. Joy Theater  thejoytheater.com, 1200 Canal St., 504-528-9569

7. Roosevelt Hotel  therooseveltneworleans.com, 130 Roosevelt Way, 504-648-1200

8. Adler's  adlersjewelry.com, 722 Canal St., 504-523-5292

9. Rubensteins  rubensteinsneworleans.com, 102 St. Charles Ave., 504-581-6666

10. The Sazerac House  sazerachouse.com, 101 Magazine St., 504-910-0100

11. Harrah's New Orleans  caesars.com/harrahs-new-orleans, 228 Poydras St., 800-427-7247

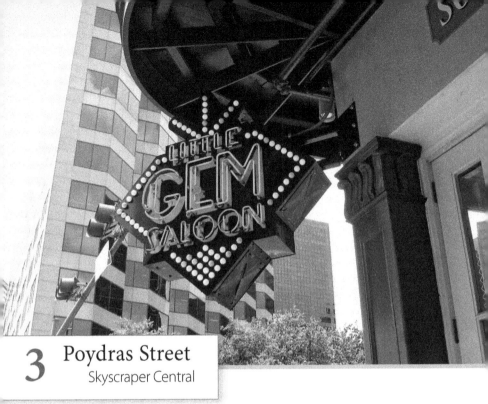

# 3 Poydras Street
## Skyscraper Central

*Above: Jazz musicians Kermit Ruffins and Shamarr Allen are among the regular performers gracing the stage at the Little Gem Saloon.*

BOUNDARIES: Mississippi River, Poydras St., S. Robertson St.
DISTANCE: 2.04 miles
PARKING: Lots, garages, metered parking
PUBLIC TRANSIT: Riverfront Streetcar, St. Charles Ave. Streetcar

Poydras Street, the main thoroughfare of the Central Business District, extends from the Mississippi River to well beyond downtown. But it's the stretch between the river and South Claiborne Avenue that serves as the heartbeat of the city's economy, with the Mercedes-Benz Superdome anchoring one side and the busy riverfront and the nearby Ernest N. Morial Convention Center the other.

Poydras Street is named after Julien Poydras, a French American politician who represented Louisiana in the US House of Representatives from 1809 to 1811. Until the oil boom of the

1980s, Poydras was just another downtown street, consisting mostly of low- to mid-rise buildings. But with the construction of the Superdome in 1975, along with such buildings as One Shell Square—the city's tallest—and 1250 Poydras Plaza, the city's skyline began taking shape. Although Poydras lost many tenants to the oil bust in the late '80s, many buildings were converted into luxury hotels to accommodate the city's ever-growing tourist industry.

Other high-rises on Poydras include the Pan American Life Center, Benson Tower, and First Bank and Trust Tower. Several hotels, restaurants, and bars can also be found on Poydras and in the surrounding business district, making New Orleans an ideal choice for conventions and big-time events such as the Super Bowl and the NCAA's Final Four. A relatively recent addition to the street is the Poydras Corridor Sculpture Exhibition, featuring more than a dozen sculptures by Southern artists, on the neutral ground between the Superdome and Convention Center Boulevard.

# Walk Description

Begin at the Hilton New Orleans Riverside and cross Poydras Street. Just across Poydras from the Hilton is the future home of city's first Four Seasons Hotel. The high-rise was once home to the World Trade Center of New Orleans and headquarters of the Port of New Orleans. Built in 1968, the 33-story structure housed foreign consulates and featured a popular revolving bar that overlooked the Mississippi River.

Turn left and continue down Poydras in front of ❶ Harrah's New Orleans, the city's only land-based casino. As of this writing, the hotel-casino was planning a major rebranding under the name Caesars New Orleans. The $352-million renovation will include a hotel, new dining options, and other amenities.

A block from the casino, at Poydras and Tchoupitoulas Streets, is ❷ Mother's Restaurant, a po'boy joint that attracts huge lunch crowds. For the uninitiated, po'boys are similar to submarine sandwiches but are made on Louisiana's famous crisp French bread. At one time, Mother's was *the* quintessential spot to grab a sloppy roast beef or fried shrimp, and while it's still worth the stop, po'boys of all sizes, fillings, and prices abound across the metro area.

Along Poydras Street, you'll pass numerous hotels and skyscrapers, including One Shell Square, between St. Charles Avenue and Carondelet Street. At 51 stories, One Shell Square is the tallest building in New Orleans and Louisiana. When it was built in 1972, it was also the tallest building in the Southeast, and the first Southern skyscraper to exceed 600 feet.

Between South Rampart Street and O'Keefe Avenue sits a mini–entertainment area featuring ❸ Copper Vine Wine Pub, ❹ Walk-On's Bistreaux & Bar, and ❺ Little Gem Saloon, a music venue with an especially fascinating history: the club actually dates back to 1904, when it served as a popular hangout for such jazz legends as Jelly Roll Morton and Buddy Bolden. It closed in 1909, and though several other businesses occupied the space over the years, the building sat dormant for nearly 40 years until a group of developers and jazz aficionados brought it back to life as Little Gem in 2012. Regular performers include Dr. Michael White's Quartet, Kermit Ruffins and the Barbecue Swingers, Trombone Shorty, and the Viper Mad Trio.

Cross Loyola Avenue and continue walking along Poydras, past the back of New Orleans City Hall and several other buildings, including 1555 Poydras, one of many buildings that make up Tulane University's downtown Health Sciences Campus.

Make a left across Poydras at South Robertson Street, and take in the wonder that is the ⑥ Superdome, among the most recognizable structures in New Orleans. Home of the New Orleans Saints since 1975, the Superdome is also home to the annual Allstate Sugar Bowl; the R&L Carriers New Orleans Bowl; the Bayou Classic; and the Essence Festival, the world's largest African American music festival. Over the years, it has undergone numerous facelifts, but none as sizable as the one following Hurricane Katrina in August 2005, when the Superdome served as a last-resort shelter for thousands of evacuees. The powerful storm peeled off part of the roof, and the damage from flooding was so extensive that the building had to be shut down for more than a year for repairs. That year, the Saints played their home games at Tiger Stadium in Baton Rouge, about 90 miles upriver from New Orleans. The Superdome reopened to much fanfare in September 2006, when the Saints beat the Atlanta Falcons in a nationally televised prime-time game.

Continue walking down Poydras to LaSalle Street. To the right, down LaSalle, is Champions Square, a festival and concert venue built after the Saints won the Super Bowl in 2010. Saints fans, donning their black and gold, enjoy partying at the Square before each home game.

Across from the Superdome is the 26-story Benson Tower, an office building owned by Saints and New Orleans Pelicans owner Gayle Benson. The Hyatt Regency New Orleans, which was shuttered for six years after Katrina, is on that same block. The Hyatt is home to ⑦ Borgne, an upscale Louisiana seafood eatery, and Vitascope Hall, a sports bar that offers both seafood and sushi. At the corner of Poydras and Loyola is a 40,000-square-foot Dave & Buster's restaurant and arcade.

Cross Loyola. To the right, on the median, is the Richard and Annette Bloch Cancer Survivors Plaza, one of two dozen parks around the country established by Richard Bloch, cofounder of H&R Block and a cancer survivor himself until his death from heart failure in 2004. The building at Loyola and Poydras is the Energy Centre, which at 39 stories is the city's fourth-tallest structure.

Between O'Keefe Avenue and Baronne Street, you'll pass a strip that includes several restaurants, including ⑧ Johnny Sánchez, a taqueria owned, in part, by Mexican American chef Aarón

Sánchez, a judge on the culinary competition series *MasterChef* on Fox. ❾ Reginelli's Pizzeria, a local chain with nine locations, is just next door.

Just behind this stretch, between Baronne and Loyola, is South Market District, a complex of luxury apartments, entertainment venues, restaurants, and shops. It is not included as part of this walk, but feel free to take a quick detour by turning right on O'Keefe. The area includes such restaurants as ❿ Maypop, a Southern-Asian fusion eatery, and ⓫ Willa Jean, a restaurant and bakery whose chef-owner Kelly Fields is a James Beard Award winner for Outstanding Pastry Chef.

From Baronne, walk three blocks down Poydras to Camp Street. The ⓬ Hale Boggs Federal Building and Courthouse takes up the block between Camp and Magazine. New Orleans has long been known as a hotbed of political corruption, and this is where many elected officials, including former Louisiana governor Edwin Edwards, met their fates.

Three blocks from the Courthouse, between Tchoupitoulas and St. Peter Streets, is the ⓭ Piazza d'Italia, built in the late 1970s as a monument to the city's Italian American community. ⓮ Poydras & Peters, a restaurant housed in the Lowe's Hotel, pays homage to the Poydras Market of 1938, which featured local seafood and produce. Pan-seared redfish and fried catfish tacos are among the items on its menu.

Walk another block to Fulton Street. Closed to traffic, Fulton is an entertainment mall featuring such restaurants as ⓯ Grand Isle and ⓰ Ruth's Chris Steak House, along with the upscale bowling alley—yes, upscale—⓱ Fulton Alley. Every winter, Harrah's New Orleans Casino (soon to be Caesars New Orleans) presents "Miracle on Fulton Street," converting the walkway into a wonderland of lights, decorations, and snowfall.

Walk another block to Convention Center Boulevard and back to the Hilton. If you're hungry, grab a bite at ⓲ Drago's Seafood, an iconic restaurant famous for its succulent chargrilled oysters.

## Points of Interest

❶ Harrah's New Orleans  caesars.com/harrahs-new-orleans, 228 Poydras St., 800-427-7247

❷ Mother's Restaurant  mothersrestaurant.net, 401 Poydras St., 504-523-9656

❸ Copper Vine Wine Pub  coppervinewine.com, 1001 Poydras St., 504-208-9535

❹ Walk-On's Bistreaux & Bar  walk-ons.com, 1009 Poydras St., 504-309-6530

❺ Little Gem Saloon  littlegemsaloon.com, 445 S. Rampart St., 504-267-4863

❻ Superdome  mbsuperdome.com, 1500 Sugar Bowl Drive, 504-587-3663

❼ Borgne  borgnerestaurant.com, 601 Loyola Ave., 504-613-3860

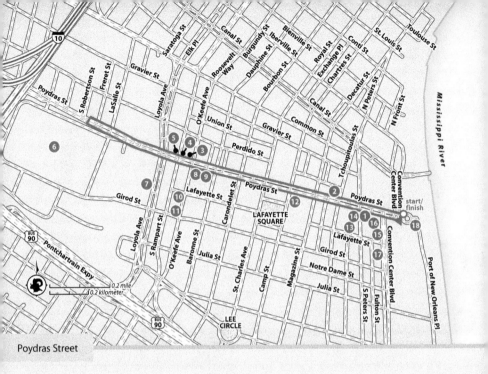

## Poydras Street

8 Johnny Sánchez New Orleans  johnnysancheznola.com, 930 Poydras St., 504-304-6615

9 Reginelli's  reginellis.com, 930 Poydras St., 504-586-0068

10 Maypop  maypoprestaurant.com, 611 O'Keefe Ave., 504-518-6345

11 Willa Jean  willajean.com, 611 O'Keefe Ave., 504-509-7334

12 Hale Boggs Federal Building and Courthouse  511-527 Poydras St.

13 Piazza d'Italia  377 Poydras St.

14 Poydras & Peters  poydrasandpeters.com, 300 Poydras St., 504-595-3305

15 Grand Isle Restaurant  grandislerestaurant.com, 575 Convention Center Blvd., 504-520-8530

16 Ruth's Chris Steak House  ruthschris.com, 525 Fulton St., 504-587-7099

17 Fulton Alley  fultonalley.com, 600 Fulton St., 504-208-5569

18 Drago's Seafood Restaurant  dragosrestaurant.com, 2 Poydras St., 504-584-3911

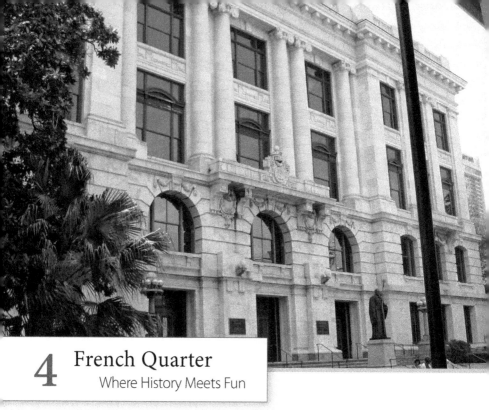

# 4 French Quarter
## Where History Meets Fun

---

*Above: The Louisiana Supreme Court Building is a Beaux Arts structure dating back to the early 1900s.*

BOUNDARIES: Iberville St., Bourbon St., St. Ann St., Decatur St.
DISTANCE: 1.66 miles
PARKING: Several garages and lots along N. Peters St.
PUBLIC TRANSIT: Riverfront Streetcar, St. Charles Ave. Streetcar

---

To much of the outside world, the French Quarter is synonymous with Bourbon Street, that often sleazy yet strangely magical playground where you can let loose with a Hurricane or a Hand Grenade, go crazy for a pair of beads, or party so hard that when you wake up the next day, you just might wonder who you are and where you've been.

But the French Quarter, or the Vieux Carré, as it's known in French, is a hotbed of fascinating history, culinary artistry, and mesmerizing music. It's the antiques shops of Royal Street, the artists of Jackson Square, and the jazz musicians of Preservation Hall. It's Friday lunch at Galatoire's or late-night drinks at the Napoleon House.

The French Quarter is the oldest neighborhood in New Orleans, developed after the city's founding in 1718 by Jean-Baptiste Le Moyne de Bienville. Most of the historic buildings in the Quarter were built in the late 18th century, after two devastating fires destroyed most of the old French Colonial architecture. At the time, New Orleans was under Spanish rule, so much of what you'll see—from wrought-iron balconies to common-wall brick houses—reflects that period.

There's so much to do and see in the Quarter that just one walking tour wouldn't do it justice. Therefore, we offer three separate walks: this one, along with the Back of the Quarter (Walk 5) and French Market/Riverfront (Walk 6).

## Walk Description

Begin at North Peters and Iberville Streets. Walk four blocks down Iberville. In the fourth block, you'll pass several classic eateries: ❶ Dickie Brennan's Steakhouse, ❷ Acme Oyster House, ❸ Bourbon House, and ❹ Felix's. At Acme and Felix's you can take in the fine art of oyster shucking while enjoying an ice-cold beer. Dickie Brennan's Steakhouse and Bourbon House are both run by restaurateur Dickie Brennan, who, with other members of the Brennan family, owns some of the city's top restaurants.

Turn right on Bourbon and brace yourself for the adult-themed playground that lies ahead. Ironically, one of the city's most critically acclaimed restaurants, the legendary ❺ Galatoire's, is among the first places you'll pass. Galatoire's dates back to 1905, when Jean Galatoire brought his culinary talents to New Orleans from the village of Pardies, France. Known for its French Creole cooking, Galatoire's boasts such dishes as crabmeat Sardou, chicken Clemenceau, oysters Rockefeller, and shrimp rémoulade. Eating at Galatoire's is the ultimate fine-dining experience, with tuxedoed waiters tending to your every need. If you're a regular, you likely have your own waiter. Although reservations are taken for the second floor, waiting in line for the more festive first floor—especially on Fridays—is the way to have a true Galatoire's experience.

Continue down Bourbon, where you'll pass strip joints, T-shirt shops, daiquiri shops, and the like. At the end of the block at Bienville Street is ❻ Jean Lafitte's Old Absinthe House, which opened its doors in 1807. Legend has it that the pirate Jean Lafitte and Andrew Jackson met on the second floor to plan the victory of the Battle of New Orleans. Over the years, the tavern has hosted such celebrities as Frank Sinatra, Mark Twain, and Liza Minnelli. Its interior features antique chandeliers and the jerseys of football legends hanging from the exposed cypress beams.

Just off the route on Bienville Street are two of the city's most popular restaurants, ❼ GW Fins and ❽ Arnaud's. Fins is known for serving fish from across the globe, and the menu changes daily based on available catch. Fins chef Tenney Flynn is so knowledgeable about seafood that he was referred to as "the fishmonger czar of the South" by the *Wall Street Journal*. Arnaud's, which dates back to 1918, is a fine-dining French establishment that, in addition to its award-winning menu, has its own Mardi Gras museum. The Germaine Cazenave Wells Mardi Gras Museum, named for the daughter of the original owner, Count Arnaud, features vintage photographs, memorabilia, and costumes that Wells and other family members wore as part of Mardi Gras royalty.

In the next block, the ⑨ Royal Sonesta Hotel is to the right. The Sonesta has long been one of the Crescent City's finest hotels. It's home to ⑩ Restaurant R'evolution, a joint venture of chefs John Folse and Rick Tramonto, who describe their fare as modern, imaginative reinterpretations of classic Cajun and Creole cuisine. Also at the Sonesta is the ⑪ Jazz Playhouse, which showcases some of the city's top jazz musicians. One of the most famous traditions associated with the Sonesta occurs every Mardi Gras, when those lucky enough to book balcony rooms arm themselves with beads to toss to the raucous revelers below. The celebrating begins the Friday before Mardi Gras (Fat Tuesday) with the annual "Greasing of the Poles," a Sonesta-sponsored event in which celebrity greasers spread petroleum jelly on the hotel's supporting poles to prevent partiers from climbing up to the balcony.

Over the next few blocks you'll pass several more bars and lounges, among them Rick's Cabaret, one of Bourbon Street's fancier strip clubs; the ⑫ Famous Door, where pianist, singer, and actor Harry Connick Jr. played his first gig at 13 years old; and the ⑬ Chris Owens Club, a burlesque joint whose ageless namesake is a French Quarter nightlife legend.

The Four Points by Sheraton French Quarter, at 541 Bourbon, occupies the one-time site of the legendary French Opera House, which served as the center of the city's social and cultural life, especially among the Creoles. The Opera House opened in 1859, and New Orleans quickly became known as "the Opera Capital of North America." It remained that way until 1919, when a fire destroyed the building.

At the corner of Bourbon and Toulouse Streets is ⑭ Tropical Isle, known for a drink called the Hand Grenade, a melon-flavored concoction that, with its mixture of "liqueurs and other secret ingredients," is billed as "New Orleans's most powerful drink." Farther down the block, to the left, is ⑮ Channing Tatum's Saints and Sinners, the bordello-themed restaurant and bar that Tatum, a regular visitor to New Orleans, opened with a business partner in 2012.

From Toulouse, walk one block to St. Peter Street and turn right. On this block, you'll pass two of the city's most beloved landmarks: ⑯ Preservation Hall and ⑰ Pat O'Brien's. Preservation Hall opened in 1961 to honor traditional New Orleans jazz. Nightly performances feature bands made up of such musicians as Gregg Stafford, Charlie Gabriel, and Wendell Brunious. All ages are welcome, so if you have children in tow, bring them along for this one-of-a-kind learning experience.

Pat O'Brien's, or Pat O's for short, is a playground within itself, an entertainment mecca since 1933, when, at the end of Prohibition, Pat O'Brien converted his speakeasy to a legal drinking establishment. Pat O's features several bars, among them a patio bar and a piano bar, where dueling entertainers lead sing-alongs from two copper-topped baby grand pianos. The signature drink is the Hurricane, a rum-based libation served in a 26-ounce souvenir glass.

Walk one block to Royal Street and turn right. Royal is the antithesis of Bourbon: a ritzy shopping stretch lined with art galleries, jewelry stores, boutiques, and antiques shops, including ⓲ M.S. Rau Antiques, which opened its doors as a small shop in 1912 and is now a 40,000-square-foot gallery overflowing with paintings and sculpture dating back to the 16th century.

At 533 Royal, between St. Louis and Toulouse Streets, is the ⓳ Historic New Orleans Collection, a museum and research center dedicated to the study and preservation of the history and culture of New Orleans and the Gulf South region. The museum's holdings include more than 35,000 library items; more than 2 miles of documents and manuscripts; and about 350,000 photographs, prints, drawings, paintings, and other artifacts. The updated and interactive Louisiana History Galleries comprises 13 galleries tracing Louisiana's fascinating past.

Walk one block to 400 Royal. The stunning Beaux Arts structure to the left is the home of the ⓴ Louisiana Supreme Court. The state's highest court moved into the building in 1910, where it remained for nearly 50 years. After the court moved to the more contemporary Central Business District, the building fell into disrepair, but it saw new life in 2004 when, after a major renovation, the supreme court returned to its Royal Street address.

Across the street is ㉑ Brennan's, the old-line restaurant renowned for its sumptuous breakfasts, world-famous bananas Foster, and romantic courtyard. To the dismay of foodies everywhere, Brennan's shut down in the summer of 2013 after its owners declared bankruptcy, but a cousin, New Orleans restaurateur Ralph Brennan, came to the rescue: he purchased the property at auction, bought back the Brennan's name, and reopened the French Quarter institution in November 2014.

In the next block, at 334 Royal St., is the headquarters of the ㉒ New Orleans Police Department's Eighth District. Erected in 1826 as the Old Bank of Louisiana, the building served as Louisiana's state capitol from 1868 to 1869, and later the Royal Street Auction Exchange and the Mortgage and Conveyance Office. This block of Royal also contains lots of fun shops, including ㉓ Vintage 329, which specializes in autographed memorabilia, rare books, and other historical items.

If you need a break—or even if you don't—stop in at the venerable Hotel Monteleone (214 Royal St.), which boasts live entertainment and one of the most popular hotel bars in New Orleans. The ㉔ Carousel Bar & Lounge features a 25-seat revolving bar with a carousel top, antiqued mirrors, and hand-painted chairs. The lounge, with its circular glass chandeliers and expansive windows along Royal Street, is equally inviting.

Turn left on Iberville Street, walk one block to Chartres Street, and turn left. Like Royal, Chartres offers a lot in the way of shopping, but it also has much to offer in the way of eating. Over the last few years, Chartres has become something of a culinary corridor, with such restaurants as **25** Justine, **26** SoBou, **27** Kingfish, **28** Doris Metropolitan, **29** Sylvain, and **30** Tableau lining the five blocks between Iberville and St. Peter Streets.

Of course, you may just opt for the **31** Napoleon House (500 Chartres St.), which has been serving up its famous Pimm's Cups and muffulettas since 1914. The Napoleon House—one of the best bars in America, according to *Esquire* magazine—is housed in a 200-year-old building that belonged to Nicolas Girod, mayor of New Orleans from 1812 to 1815. Girod offered his residence to Napoleon Bonaparte in 1821 as a refuge during his exile; alas, Napoleon died before he could make it to New Orleans.

A few doors down from the Napoleon House is the **32** Pharmacy Museum (514 Chartres St.), the one-time apothecary shop of Louis Joseph Dufilho Jr., who in the early 19th century became America's first licensed pharmacist. On display are old patent medicines, books, and pharmaceutical equipment dating back as far as the early 1800s, as well as surgical instruments used in the Civil War. Other exhibits include a re-created 19th-century physician's study and a spectacle collection illustrating the historical development of eyewear and other antique vision aids from around the world.

Continue walking to the corner of Chartres and St. Peter Streets. To your left is **33** Le Petit Théâtre du Vieux Carré, one of the oldest community theaters in the country. Originally organized in 1916 as the New Orleans Chapter of the Drama League of America, the company began performing in this space in 1922. The theater has undergone numerous renovations, including the addition of Tableau, a Dickie Brennan restaurant specializing in Louisiana Creole fare.

Continue walking on Chartres straight into Jackson Square, the highlight of which is the triple-spired **34** St. Louis Cathedral, the oldest cathedral in North America and easily the city's most recognizable landmark. The church features a Rococo-style gilded altar along with magnificent stained glass windows and paintings. In the rear of the cathedral is the St. Anthony Garden, where a statue of Jesus stands with arms upraised. Stop in for Mass or a tour; the cathedral is open daily after the 7:30 a.m. Mass until 4 p.m., and self-guided tours are available for a $1 donation.

The cathedral is flanked by the **35** Cabildo and the **36** Presbytère, two of several museums under the Louisiana State Museum umbrella. Facing the cathedral, the Cabildo is to your left. Built in the late 18th century, the Cabildo served as the seat of government in New Orleans during the Spanish Colonial period and is where the Louisiana Purchase—which nearly doubled the size of the United States—was signed in 1803. To your right is the Presbytère, a one-time courthouse that now houses an exquisite collection of Mardi Gras artifacts and memorabilia. Through an interactive exhibit titled *Mardi Gras: It's Carnival Time in Louisiana,* visitors can learn the history of Mardi Gras, from its 19th-century beginnings to the modern-day celebration that attracts millions of tourists every year.

Though not on the walk, ❸❼ **Faulkner House Books** (624 Pirate's Alley), once the home of legendary writer William Faulkner, is worth a stop. Stroll down Pirate's Alley, between the Cabildo and St. Louis Cathedral, and you'll find it.

Take your time strolling around ❸❽ **Jackson Square**, enjoying the vibrancy of the artists, musicians, and other street performers at work. The redbrick buildings on either side of the square are the Lower and Upper Pontalba Buildings, the oldest apartments in the United States. The apartments take up the top three stories, while shops and restaurants occupy the first. One of the best of the eateries is ❸❾ **Stanley**, at the corner of St. Ann and Chartres, a casual café known for its all-day breakfast fare. Another restaurant worth checking out is ❹⓿ **Muriel's Jackson Square**, just across Chartres from Stanley. Muriel's serves contemporary Creole fare and boasts one of the best dining balconies in town.

If you have a few extra minutes to spare, walk through the square, named for General Andrew Jackson, the hero of the Battle of New Orleans. Known in the 18th century as the Place d'Armes, the historic park is a popular site for television broadcasts and music festivals, including the French Quarter Festival and Caroling in the Square.

Continue around the square along Decatur Street, across from Café Du Monde, the famous coffee-and-beignets stand. This block of Decatur is an assembly spot for horse-drawn-carriage tours. Walk to St. Peter Street, turn right, and head one more block back to Chartres Street. The tour ends here, but be sure to check out the Back of the Quarter and the French Market/Riverfront area, each covered in the next two walks.

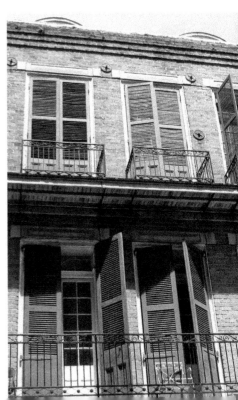

*Balconied apartment buildings such as this one can be found throughout the French Quarter.*

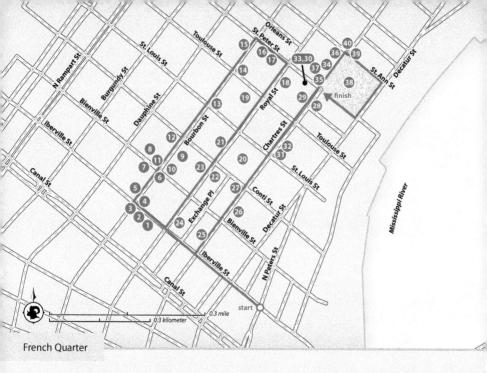

French Quarter

## Points of Interest

1. Dickie Brennan's Steakhouse  dickiebrennanssteakhouse.com, 716 Iberville St., 504-522-2467

2. Acme Oyster House  acmeoyster.com, 724 Iberville St., 504-522-5973

3. Bourbon House  bourbonhouse.com, 144 Bourbon St., 504-522-0111

4. Felix's Restaurant and Oyster Bar  felixs.com, 739 Iberville St., 504-522-4440

5. Galatoire's  galatoires.com, 209 Bourbon St., 504-525-2021

6. Jean Lafitte's Old Absinthe House  ruebourbon.com/old-absinthe-house, 240 Bourbon St., 504-523-3181

7. GW Fins  gwfins.com, 808 Bienville St., 504-581-3467

8. Arnaud's  arnaudsrestaurant.com, 813 Bienville St., 504-523-5433

9. Royal Sonesta Hotel New Orleans  sonesta.com/royalneworleans, 300 Bourbon St., 504-586-0300

10. Restaurant R'evolution  revolutionnola.com, 777 Bienville St., 504-553-2277

11. Jazz Playhouse  sonesta.com/jazzplayhouse, 300 Bourbon St., 504-553-2299

12. Famous Door  339 Bourbon St., 504-598-4334

(13) Chris Owens Club  500 Bourbon St., 504-523-6400

(14) Tropical Isle  tropicalisle.com, 600 Bourbon St., 504-529-1702

(15) Saints and Sinners  saintsandsinnersnola.com, 627 Bourbon St., 504-528-9307

(16) Preservation Hall  preservationhall.com, 726 St. Peter St., 504-522-2841

(17) Pat O'Brien's  patobriens.com, 718 St. Peter St., 504-525-4823

(18) M.S. Rau Antiques  rauantiques.com, 622 Royal St., 888-557-2406

(19) Historic New Orleans Collection  hnoc.org, 522 Royal St., 504-523-4662

(20) Louisiana Supreme Court  lasc.org, 400 Royal St., 504-310-2300

(21) Brennan's  brennansneworleans.com, 417 Royal St., 504-525-9711

(22) New Orleans Police Department, Eighth District  nola.gov/nopd, 334 Royal St., 504-658-6080

(23) Vintage 329  vintage329.com, 329 Royal St., 504-525-2262

(24) Carousel Bar & Lounge, Hotel Monteleone  hotelmonteleone.com, 214 Royal St., 504-523-3341

(25) Justine  justinenola.com, 225 Chartres St., 504-218-8533

(26) SoBou  sobounola.com, 310 Chartres St., 504-552-4095

(27) Kingfish  kingfishneworleans.com, 337 Chartres St., 504-598-5005

(28) Doris Metropolitan  dorismetropolitan.com, 620 Chartres St., 504-267-3500

(29) Sylvain  sylvainnola.com, 625 Chartres St., 504-265-8123

(30) Tableau  tableaufrenchquarter.com, 616 St. Peter St., 504-934-3463

(31) Napoleon House  napoleonhouse.com, 500 Chartres St., 504-524-9752

(32) Pharmacy Museum  pharmacymuseum.org, 514 Chartres St., 504-565-8027

(33) Le Petit Théâtre du Vieux Carré  lepetittheatre.com, 616 St. Peter St., 504-522-2081

(34) St. Louis Cathedral  stlouiscathedral.org, Jackson Square, 504-525-9585

(35) The Cabildo  crt.state.la.us/louisiana-state-museum, 701 Chartres St., 504-568-6968

(36) The Presbytère  crt.state.la.us/louisiana-state-museum, 751 Chartres St., 504-568-6968

(37) Faulkner House Books  faulknerhousebooks.com, 624 Pirates Alley, 504-524-2940

(38) Jackson Square  nola.gov/parks-and-parkways/parks-squares/jackson-square, bounded by St. Ann, St. Peter, Decatur, and Chartres Streets; 504-658-3200

(39) Stanley  stanleyrestaurant.com, 547 St. Ann St., 504-587-0093

(40) Muriel's Jackson Square  muriels.com, 801 Chartres St., 504-568-1885

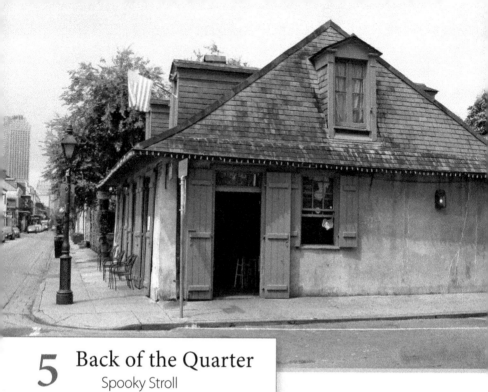

## 5 Back of the Quarter
### Spooky Stroll

---

*Above: Lafitte's Blacksmith Shop is believed to be the oldest structure used as a bar in the United States.*

---

BOUNDARIES: Esplanade Ave., Chartres St., Dumaine St., Dauphine St.
DISTANCE: 1.73 miles
PARKING: Limited street parking
PUBLIC TRANSIT: RTA Bus #5 (Marigny-Bywater), Riverfront Streetcar

---

The French Quarter isn't all about Bourbon Street. In fact, the lower part of the Quarter, between Esplanade Avenue and St. Ann Street, is a mostly residential neighborhood where homes range from restored Creole cottages to French Colonial town houses sporting exquisite wrought-iron balconies. It's relatively quiet, but no less fascinating or historic than its more popular counterpart upriver.

Many of the homes in the Lower French Quarter have been converted to museums, giving visitors an up-close view of 18th- and 19th-century lifestyles; among the more notable examples are the Beauregard-Keyes House and the Gallier House. Some of the city's allegedly haunted houses—like the legendary LaLaurie House—can be found here as well. Even the hotels and inns, such as the Soniat House and the Cornstalk Hotel, have historic significance.

Of course, no New Orleans neighborhood is complete without a culinary component, and two of the best are Café Amelie, a French eatery that boasts one of the city's most delightful outdoor dining areas, and just down the block, Petite Amelie, where the "cuisine rapide" menu includes salads, sandwiches, and light breakfast fare. For po'boys, check out Verti Marte. For libations, Harry's Corner and Lafitte's Blacksmith Shop are among the classics.

# Walk Description

Begin at the ❶ New Orleans Jazz Museum at the Old US Mint (Esplanade Avenue at North Peters Street), one of several museums that make up the Louisiana State Museum system. Built in 1835, the Greek Revival building served as a mint for both the Union and the Confederacy. Today, it's home to exhibits on Louis Prima, Professor Longhair, and other New Orleans jazz greats. The museum also hosts a regular series of jazz performances.

Walk two blocks to Chartres Street and turn left. At 1133 Chartres is the ❷ Soniat House, built in the 1820s by Joseph Soniat Dufossat, a French sugar plantation owner. Now a boutique hotel, the property consists of three town houses with 31 guest rooms furnished and decorated with French and English antiques. It has won many accolades, among them being named one of the top 20 hotels in the world by Fodor's.

Continue down Chartres. At the end of the block is the ❸ Beauregard-Keyes House, a raised center-hall house built in 1826 by architect François Correjolles for auctioneer Joseph LeCarpentier. The house had a number of notable residents over the years, including 19th-century chess master Paul Morphy and Confederate general P. G. T. Beauregard, who rented it from 1866 to 1868 after the Civil War. Novelist Frances Parkinson Keyes, who wrote such historical fiction as *Madame Castel's Lodger* and *Blue Camellia*, lived here from 1945 until her death in 1970. Keyes, with the help of architect Sam Wilson, restored the house and established the Keyes Foundation, which maintains it to this day. The house reflects the years that Beauregard lived there and features furniture and art owned by the general and his family, along with Keyes's writing studio and her extensive collections of dolls and porcelain.

Across the street is the ❹ Old Ursuline Convent, the oldest building in the Mississippi Valley, having been designed and constructed over an eight-year period from 1745 to 1753. The building has served several purposes over the centuries, from convent and school to archbishop's residence and central office of the Archdiocese of New Orleans. It is now the home of the Catholic Cultural Heritage Center.

Continue down Chartres to St. Philip Street.

In the next block, at the corner of Chartres and Dumaine, is ❺ Harry's Corner, treasured by those looking for a French Quarter bar experience away from the craziness of Bourbon Street.

Walk one more block to Dumaine Street and turn right. At 632 Dumaine is ❻ Madame John's Legacy, a complex of 18th-century Louisiana Creole buildings that escaped the Great New Orleans Fire of 1794. Designed in the French West Indies style, it encompasses three buildings: the main house, which is open to the public; the kitchen; and the two-story gentlemen's guest quarters.

Walk to the end of the block and turn right on Royal Street. At 900, 906, and 910 Royal are the ❼ Miltenberger Houses, a row of three town houses built in the 1830s by Marie Miltenberger, a widow whose husband, Dr. Christian Miltenberger, had been renowned for his work with yellow fever patients. The houses, with their cast-iron galleries and floor-to-ceiling windows, are among the most photographed in the Quarter. Next door, at 912 Royal, is ❽ Café Amelie, a French restaurant with what restaurant critic Brett Anderson called "one of the city's most romantic outdoor settings." For a quick bite, ❾ Petite Amelie is just down the block.

Across the street at 915 Royal St. is the ❿ Cornstalk Hotel, famous for its cast-iron fence depicting ears of corn intertwined with morning glories. The hotel was built as a residence for Judge François Xavier Martin, chief justice of the Louisiana Supreme Court, who lived there from 1816 to 1826. Dr. Joseph Secondo Biamenti bought the mansion in 1834, converted it to a hotel, and added its famous fence. Prominent guests include Bill and Hillary Clinton, Elvis Presley, and Harriet Beecher Stowe, who used nearby slave quarters as her inspiration for *Uncle Tom's Cabin*.

Walk two blocks to 1132 Royal St., the residence of noted architect James Gallier and his family during the mid-19th century. The ⓫ Gallier House, which is open to the public, tells the story of those who lived and worked on the property. In addition to the home itself, the tour ($15 adults, $12 seniors and kids) includes the gardens, carriageway, and restored slave quarters. The house is especially fun to visit in December, when it's embellished in holiday dress.

Just down the block, at 1140 Royal St., is the ⓬ LaLaurie House—also known simply as "the Haunted House"—which, along with its evil owner, was featured in the FX series *American Horror Story: Coven.* Madame Delphine LaLaurie, a wealthy socialite, bought the Creole mansion in 1831, and incredible stories of wild parties and servant abuse soon followed. When a fire broke out in 1834, neighbors broke in through a locked door and found seven slaves chained and starving. As outraged citizens protested outside, a carriage sped into the crowd and away from the premises;

in the carriage were Madame LaLaurie and her family, who escaped to Paris, never to return. Legend has it that the spirits of the slaves still inhabit the mansion, making it a favorite stop on haunted-history tours.

Turn left on Governor Nicholls Street. At the corner of Governor Nicholls and Royal is the ⑬ Verti Marte, a beloved French Quarter institution known for its All That Jazz po'boy (sautéed shrimp, turkey, ham, mushrooms, Swiss and American cheeses, and a special "Wow Sauce"). The place is open 24 hours a day, seven days a week, making it wildly popular with locals.

Walk one block to Bourbon Street and turn left. Walk two blocks to ⑭ Lafitte's Blacksmith Shop (941 Bourbon St.), a tavern that was built between 1722 and 1732 and is considered one of the oldest structures used as a bar in the United States. According to Lafitte's website, the property is believed to have been used by pirates Jean and Pierre Lafitte as a New Orleans base for their smuggling operation.

Walk two blocks to 739 Bourbon St., home of ⑮ Marie Laveau's House of Voodoo. Named for the city's most famous voodoo queen, this fun souvenir shop sells everything from tribal masks and statues to voodoo dolls and spell kits. And if you want to have your palm read or your fortune told, you're at the right place.

Head right on St. Ann Street (left if you're leaving the House of Voodoo), walk one block to Dauphine Street, then turn right and take Dauphine five blocks to Esplanade Avenue. At the corner of St. Ann and Dauphine, on your left, you'll pass ⑯ Good Friends Bar, one of the city's most popular gay bars. Farther up Dauphine, you'll also pass ⑰ Cabrini Playground on your left, between Governor Nicholls and Barracks Streets. Yes, there is an actual playground in the French Quarter (along with two schools), because families with young children really do live here.

Turn right on Esplanade Avenue. As you round the corner, don't be surprised to see a crowd of people standing in front of 838 Esplanade—this is ⑱ Port of Call, which, even with the proliferation of burger restaurants across town, is considered one of the city's best.

Walk five blocks back to your starting point at the New Orleans Jazz Museum at the Old US Mint.

## Points of Interest

① New Orleans Jazz Museum at the Old US Mint  crt.state.la.us, 400 Esplanade Ave., 504-568-2022
② Soniat House  soniathouse.com, 1133 Chartres St., 504-522-0570
③ Beauregard-Keyes House  bkhouse.org, 1113 Chartres St., 504-523-7257
④ Old Ursuline Convent  oldursulineconventmuseum.com, 1100 Chartres St., 504-529-3040

*(continued on next page)*

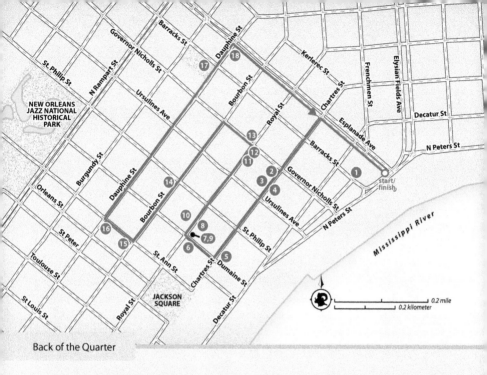

Back of the Quarter

*(continued from previous page)*

5. Harry's Corner  900 Chartres St., 504-524-1107

6. Madame John's Legacy  crt.state.la.us/louisiana-state-museum, 632 Dumaine St., 504-568-6968

7. Miltenberger Houses  900, 906, and 910 Royal St.

8. Café Amelie  cafeamelie.com, 912 Royal St., 504-412-8965

9. Petite Amelie  petiteamelienola.wordpress.com, 900 Royal St., 504-412-8065

10. Cornstalk Hotel  cornstalkhotel.com, 915 Royal St., 504-523-1515

11. Gallier House  hgghh.org, 1132 Royal St., 504-525-5661

12. LaLaurie House  1140 Royal St.

13. Verti Marte  1201 Royal St., 504-525-4767

14. Lafitte's Blacksmith Shop  lafittesblacksmithshop.com, 941 Bourbon St., 504-593-9761

15. Marie Laveau's House of Voodoo  voodooneworleans.com, 739 Bourbon St., 504-581-3751

16. Good Friends Bar  goodfriendsbar.com, 740 Dauphine St., 504-566-7191

17. Cabrini Playground  Dauphine Street between Governor Nicholls and Barracks Streets

18. Port of Call  portofcallnola.com, 838 Esplanade Ave., 504-523-0120

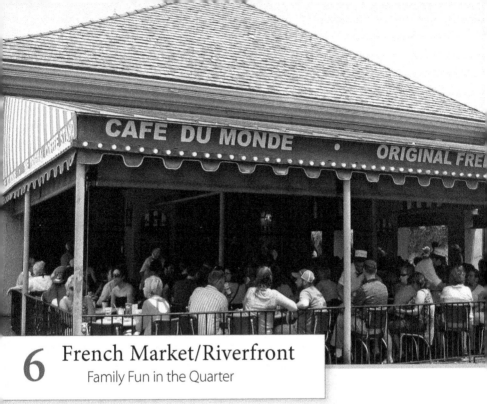

# 6 French Market/Riverfront
## Family Fun in the Quarter

---

*Above: A visit to New Orleans wouldn't be complete without a trip to Café Du Monde, famous for its sugar-dusted beignets and café au lait.*

---

BOUNDARIES: Bienville St., Decatur St., Barracks St., Mississippi River
DISTANCE: 1.62 miles
PARKING: Several parking lots along Decatur
PUBLIC TRANSIT: Riverfront Streetcar, RTA Buses #5 (Marigny-Bywater) and #55 (Elysian Fields)

---

The Riverfront area between Canal Street and Esplanade Avenue may be part of the French Quarter, but it's also a world within itself: a vibrant mix of attractions that includes the lively French Market, a riverfront promenade, and a linear park with lush pathways and stunning sculptures.

Founded in 1791, the French Market is the oldest public market in the United States. Stretching six blocks from Barracks Street to St. Ann Street, it was established as a Native American trading post and at one time was the only legal place in the city to buy meat. Its latest incarnation is that of a culinary corridor complete with countertop dining, a cooking-demonstration stage, and live musical performances.

Other focal points of the area include the Moon Walk, a riverfront walkway with spectacular views; Woldenberg Park, among the treasures of the Audubon Nature Institute; and the world-famous Café Du Monde, which has been serving café au lait and sugar-laden beignets since 1862.

Annual festivals add to the frivolity of the Riverfront, including the French Quarter Festival, the Creole Tomato Festival, the Bastille Day Fête, and the Mighty Mississippi River Festival. If you have kids in tow, bring them along—the French Quarter, at least this part of it, truly is a family destination.

## Walk Description

Begin your walk in front of ❶ Monty's on the Square, a restaurant at the corner of Decatur and St. Ann Streets in Jackson Square. Walk upriver, away from the square, to 923 Decatur St., home of ❷ Central Grocery, a small Italian market where the famous muffuletta was invented by founder Salvatore Lupo, a Sicilian immigrant, back in 1906. The muffuletta is a sandwich made with round Italian bread and stuffed with cold cuts, cheese, and olive salad. In addition to Italian delicacies, the market sells a variety of French, Spanish, Greek, and Creole specialty foods. Stop in, if only to take a whiff.

Continue walking down Decatur, where you'll pass numerous souvenir and T-shirt shops, including one called ❸ Jazz Funeral, which, with merchandise like skeletons and voodoo dolls, is in keeping with the haunted lore of the Quarter. In the block between Ursulines Avenue and Governor Nicholls Street, you'll pass ❹ B.B. King's Blues Club, part of a national chain of soulful blues clubs; ❺ Molly's at the Market, the city's unofficial media bar, and ❻ Coop's Place, a great place to grab some grub after a night at Molly's. ❼ Cane & Table is known for its rum-inspired drinks and island-themed fare.

In the next block, to your right, is the ❽ Palm Court Jazz Cafe, where you can listen to traditional New Orleans jazz while dining on such Louisiana fare as red beans and rice, crawfish pie, and Creole gumbo. Nina Buck and her late husband, jazz musician George Buck, opened Palm Court in 1989 in a fully restored early-19th-century building. In addition to the Palm Court Jazz Band, regular performers include Clive Wilson's New Orleans Serenaders, the Crescent City Joymakers, and musicians Mark Braud and Lars Edegran. Trumpeter Lionel Ferbos, the Palm Court Jazz Band's longtime front man, was considered New Orleans's oldest working musician. (Ferbos, who died in July 2014 at age 103, performed regularly until 2013.) Need a break? Check out ❾ EnVie Espresso Bar & Cafe for its impressive menu of coffee drinks and pastries.

# Audubon Aquarium of the Americas

From the moment you walk through the underwater tunnel at the Audubon Aquarium of the Americas, you know you've arrived at a special place. Part of the Aquarium's Caribbean Reef Exhibit, the glass-enclosed tunnel is surrounded by a 132,000-gallon tank where exotic creatures such as angelfish, cownose rays, and moray eels swim about to the delight of visitors. The tunnel is one of the Aquarium's trademark features, but it's just the beginning of a fascinating journey through the waters of the Americas, from the Amazon to the Caribbean.

The interactive *Geaux Fish!* exhibit showcases Louisiana's fishing industry and invites you to cast a virtual reel, identify local species, visit a seafood market, and board a fishing boat. *Parakeet Pointe* is an 800-square-foot outdoor area where you can meander among hundreds of vibrant parakeets and, for a minimal charge, buy seed sticks and feed the birds. *Escape Extinction: Sharks* is a family-friendly escape room, where through puzzles and games you can work in small groups to save sharks from going extinct. You can even experience the Amazon Orinoco rainforest by climbing into the Amazon "tree-top loop" and marveling at such exotic species of fish as payara piranhas, pacu fish, and freshwater stingrays. One of the aquarium's most popular sites is the Penguin Exhibit, featuring a colony of penguins from South America and Africa.

Be sure to pick up a schedule of feedings, chats, and other daily events at the information booth. And if time allows, pair your visit to the Aquarium with tickets to the Entergy IMAX Theatre just next door, where you can choose from an array of award-winning nature films. The theater's five-and-a-half-story screen—the largest IMAX screen in the Gulf South—makes for an unmatched viewing experience.

Walk to Barracks Street, turn right, and enter the back side of the ⑩ **French Market**. The market has undergone numerous changes since it opened in 1791, but one thing that hasn't changed is its status as a cultural and commercial icon. This six-block stretch includes a vibrant flea market, where vendors sell jewelry, artwork, candles, and other merchandise 365 days a year. The flea market leads to the farmers market, which has a variety of food stands, along with fresh produce, seafood, and baked goods. Eateries include Alberto's Cheese & Wine Bistro; Mother Nature's Cupboard; J's Seafood Dock; and Meals from the Heart Café, which serves vegetarian, vegan, and gluten-free fare. The guys shucking oysters are a show in themselves.

Continue walking through the French Market to Ursulines Avenue. Turn left, then turn right at North Peters Street. To your right is Latrobe Park, a lush green space where you can take a break on one of the benches and enjoy the sounds of jazz coming from the nearby Gazebo Café. Dedicated to architect Benjamin Latrobe, the park sits on the site of the city's first waterworks, which Latrobe designed. He died from yellow fever in 1820 as he was working on the project.

Walk a block to St. Philip Street. To your right is Place de France, a tiny park that houses a golden bronze statue of Joan of Arc atop a horse. The equestrian statue, a gift from France to New Orleans in 1959, is a replica of the 1880 Emmanuel Fremiet statue in the Place des Pyramides in Paris.

At this point, North Peters turns into Decatur Street. Continue walking past the myriad shops that line the next block. Stop in one of the praline shops along the way. Most are more than happy to let you sample their confections.

Walk a block to Dumaine Street. To the left is ⑪ Dutch Alley, a promenade that runs parallel to North Peters. Named for the late Mayor Ernest "Dutch" Morial, Dutch Alley is home to an artists' co-op managed and operated by nearly two dozen craftspeople. Original art on display includes jewelry, photography, paintings, pottery, fabric art, and works made from salvaged materials and glass. In the same area is the ⑫ New Orleans Jazz National Historical Park, which presents jazz performances, lectures, films, and exhibits.

At the corner of St. Ann and Decatur is ⑬ Café Du Monde, known for its café au lait (half coffee, half milk) and beignets, square pieces of dough fried and covered with powdered sugar. This is the original Café Du Monde, which opened in 1862 and continues to operate seven days a week, 24 hours a day (except on Christmas Day).

From the side of Café Du Monde, take the stairs up to ⑭ Washington Artillery Park, a raised plaza that pays homage to the 141st Field Artillery of the Louisiana National Guard, the oldest artillery unit in the United States. The park features a replica of a cannon used in the Civil War. With Jackson Square and St. Louis Cathedral on one side and the Mississippi River on the other side, this is one of the most photographed spots in New Orleans.

Take the stairs down to the ground level, and cross the parking lot and streetcar tracks to the entrance of the Moon Walk, a riverfront promenade where you can relax on a bench and enjoy the views. The Moon Walk is named for former Mayor Moon Landrieu, under whose leadership the walkway opened in the 1970s.

Once on the Moon Walk, turn right and continue walking. Among the landmarks that you'll pass are the ⑮ Shops at Jax Brewery, to your right, a shopping mall that once served as the brewhouse for Jax Beer. The four floors of stores, restaurants, bars, and attractions include the Jax Collection, a museum where you can learn the fascinating history of Jax Beer. To your left is the Toulouse Street Wharf, which serves as the entrance for the ⑯ Steamboat *Natchez*, the last authentic steamboat on the Mississippi. The *Natchez* offers a variety of jazz and dining cruises.

The Moon Walk leads to ⑰ Woldenberg Riverfront Park, named for philanthropist Malcolm Woldenberg. The 16-acre park features a jogging path along with artwork and sculptures, including a stunning Holocaust Memorial Exhibit. The park is a backdrop for the French Quarter Festival, the New Orleans Oyster Festival, and the Zulu Lundi Gras Festival, among other big-time events. It is part of the Audubon Nature Institute, which also operates the ⑱ Aquarium of the Americas (see sidebar on page 35) and the ⑲ Entergy IMAX Theatre, both of which are adjacent to the park. Exit the park via Bienville Street.

Turn right on North Peters Street and walk two blocks to Toulouse Street. North Peters becomes Decatur Street. Walk four blocks down Decatur back to your starting point. On the way, you'll pass the new location of ⑳ Tujague's, the second-oldest restaurant in New Orleans. You'll also pass ㉑ Jackson Square, where artists line the sidewalk turning blank canvasses into stunning works of art, from oil paintings to caricatures. Although it's not on this walk, ㉒ Beckham's Bookshop (228 Decatur St.) is nearby and a fun place to browse secondhand books, CDs, and record albums. The shop boasts more than 50,000 used books on two stories. It's dog friendly too.

## Points of Interest

① Monty's on the Square  montysonthesquare.com, 801 Decatur St., 504-525-4478

② Central Grocery  923 Decatur St., 504-523-1620

③ Jazz Funeral  929 Decatur St., 504-412-9561

④ B.B. King's Blues Club  bbkings.com/new-orleans, 1104 Decatur St., 504-934-5464

⑤ Molly's at the Market  mollysatthemarket.net, 1107 Decatur St., 504-525-5169

⑥ Coop's Place  coopsplace.net, 1109 Decatur St., 504-525-9053

⑦ Cane & Table  caneandtablenola.com, 1113 Decatur St., 504-581-1112

⑧ Palm Court Jazz Cafe  palmcourtjazzcafe.com, 1204 Decatur St., 504-525-0200

⑨ EnVie Espresso Bar & Cafe  cafeenvie.com, 1241 Decatur St., 504-524-3689

⑩ French Market  frenchmarket.org, 1235 N. Peters St., 504-596-3420

⑪ Dutch Alley Artist's Co-op  dutchalleyartistsco-op.com, 912 N. Peters St., 504-412-9220

⑫ New Orleans Jazz National Historical Park  nps.gov/jazz, 916 N. Peters St., 504-589-4841

⑬ Café Du Monde  cafedumonde.com, 800 Decatur St., 504-525-4544

⑭ Washington Artillery Park  washingtonartillery.com, 749 Decatur St., 504-596-3420

⑮ Shops at Jax Brewery  shopsatjaxbrewery.com, 600 Decatur St., 504-566-7245

*(continued on next page)*

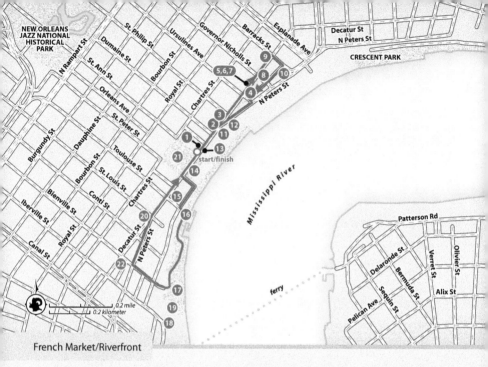

French Market/Riverfront

(continued from previous page)

16 Steamboat *Natchez* steamboatnatchez.com, Toulouse Street Wharf, 504-569-1401

17 Woldenberg Riverfront Park audubonnatureinstitute.org/woldenberg-park, 1 Canal St., 504-565-3033

18 Audubon Aquarium of the Americas audubonnatureinstitute.org/aquarium, 1 Canal St., 504-565-3033

19 Entergy IMAX Theatre audubonnatureinstitute.org/theater, 1 Canal St., 504-565-3033

20 Tujague's tujaguesrestaurant.com, 429 Decatur St., 504-525-8676

21 Jackson Square nola.gov/parks-and-parkways/parks-squares/jackson-square, bounded by St. Ann, St. Peter, Decatur, and Chartres Streets; 504-658-3200

22 Beckham's Bookshop beckhamsbookshop.com, 228 Decatur St., 504-522-9875

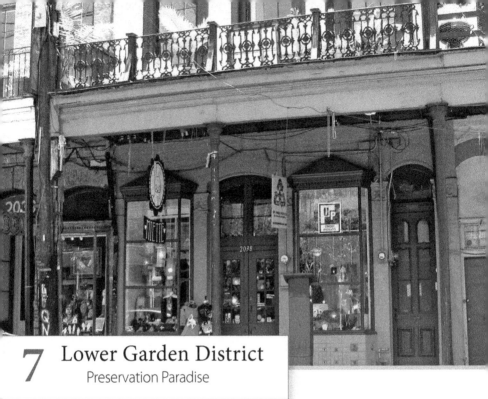

# 7 Lower Garden District
## Preservation Paradise

*Above: A stroll through the Lower Garden District will take you past some of the funkiest shops on Magazine Street, including Miette, which sells locally made jewelry, clothing, and home accessories.*

BOUNDARIES: Coliseum St., Magazine St., Josephine St., Melpomene St.
DISTANCE: 1.35 miles
PARKING: Free and metered parking
PUBLIC TRANSIT: St. Charles Ave. Streetcar

The Lower Garden District is situated just downriver from the Garden District, but the two neighborhoods are nothing alike. And that's a good thing, because it gives visitors and locals alike a chance to explore yet another area rich in history, beauty, and, in the case of the Lower Garden District, funkiness.

Developed in the early 19th century by architect Barthélemy Lafon, the Lower Garden District boasts elegant mansions that date back to the Civil War, along with a grand square and streets named after the nine muses of Greek mythology. Although the neighborhood saw its share of tough times in the mid-20th century, with many Greek Revival and Italianate mansions falling into decline, preservationists and an active neighborhood association spearheaded its comeback.

Today, the Lower Garden District is a vibrant neighborhood with a cool commercial stretch that includes restaurants, galleries, salons, boutiques, and bars. The association is as active as ever, helping maintain the area's parks and green spaces, working with police and firefighters to enhance safety, and working toward the remediation of blighted properties.

## Walk Description

Begin at Coliseum and Terpsichore Streets in front of ❶ Coliseum Square, a lush neighborhood park with live oaks, walking trails, a fountain, and benches. Facing the park, turn left and walk three blocks to Race Street. To the right, you'll pass some of the neighborhood's most exquisite homes. Among them, at 1741 Coliseum, is a double-gallery Greek Revival house built in 1847 for commission merchant Hugh Wilson. At 1749 Coliseum is the one-time home of Grace King, a Louisiana historian and author who lived there from 1905 to 1932. Built in 1847 by banker Frederick Rodewald, the Greek Revival house has both Ionic and Corinthian columns.

Turn left at Race Street and walk three blocks to Magazine Street. Turn right on Magazine in front of ❷ St. Vincent's Guest House, which was founded as St. Vincent's Infant Asylum in 1861 by the Daughters of Charity, an order of nuns. (Orphanages were a sad necessity back then because of the thousands of people who were dying from yellow fever.) St. Vincent's later became a home for unwed mothers but shut its doors in the 1970s, largely because of high operating expenses. The building remained empty until Peter Schreiber and Sally Leonard bought it, remodeled it, and opened it as a guest house in 1994.

Walk three blocks on Magazine to Felicity Street and veer right, passing ❸ Gris-Gris, a popular eatery known for Southern classics; ❹ Union Ramen, where Nhat "Chef Nate" Nguyen focuses on *tori* (poultry based) and miso (plant based); and ❺ Il Mercato, a Spanish Colonial–style building constructed in 1931 as a neighborhood market but, decades later, transformed into one of the city's most popular wedding venues.

Continue walking down Magazine past such restaurants as ❻ Garden District Pub, ❼ Pho Noi Viet, ❽ Juan's Flying Burrito, and ❾ Mayas Nuevo Latino. This stretch also features some of Magazine's most eclectic shops, including ❿ Aidan Gill for Men, an upscale men's clothing store; ⓫ Miette, a fun jewelry and gift store; and ⓬ Trashy Diva, a vintage-clothing boutique.

Turn right on Josephine Street and walk one block to Camp Street. Turn right on Camp and walk five blocks to Coliseum Square. Continue on Camp to Terpsichore. To your right is the ⓭ International School of Louisiana, a charter school founded in 2000 by a group of parents who wanted a foreign language–based academic program for their children. The school, which has two other campuses in the New Orleans area, was the state's first language-immersion charter school. In 2007, it was named a Charter School of the Year by the Center for Education Reform, the nation's leading education advocacy organization. The school emphasizes French- and Spanish-language immersion, international awareness, the celebration of diversity, and community responsibility.

Continue walking around the square to Melpomene Street. Turn left at Melpomene, then left on Coliseum and back to the starting point.

*Coliseum Square Park is surrounded by mid-19th-century mansions, such as this Greek Revival home built in 1847.*

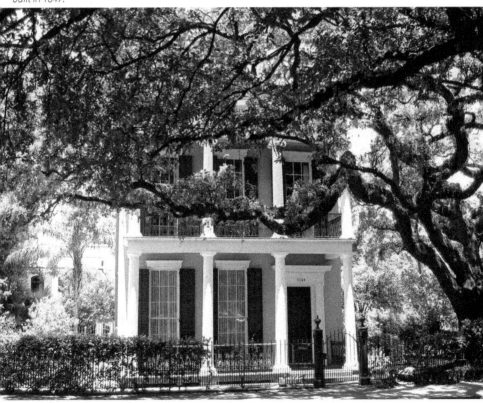

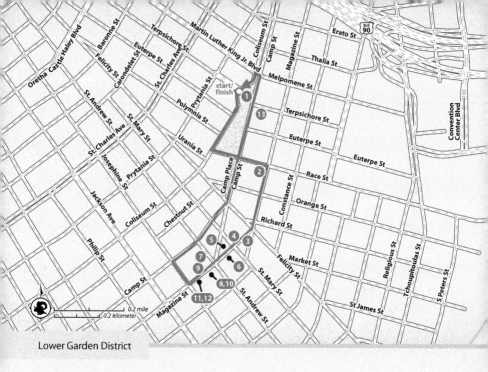

Lower Garden District

# Points of Interest

1. **Coliseum Square Park** 1700 Coliseum St.

2. **St. Vincent's Guest House** stvguesthouse.com, 1507 Magazine St., 504-302-9606

3. **Gris-Gris** grisgrisnola.com, 1800 Magazine St., 504-272-0241

4. **Union Ramen** unionramen.com, 1837 Magazine St., 504-459-2819

5. **Il Mercato** ilmercatoevents.com, 1911 Magazine St., 504-827-2400

6. **Garden District Pub** gardendistrictpub1916.com, 1916 Magazine St., 504-267-3392

7. **Pho Noi Viet** pho-noi-viet.business.site, 2005 Magazine St., 504-522-3399

8. **Juan's Flying Burrito** juansflyingburrito.com, 2018 Magazine St., 504-569-0000

9. **Mayas Nuevo Latino** 2027 Magazine St., 504-309-3401

10. **Aidan Gill for Men** aidangillformen.com, 2026 Magazine St., 504-587-9090

11. **Miette** iheartmiette.com, 2038 Magazine St., 504-522-2883

12. **Trashy Diva** trashydiva.com, 2048 Magazine St., 504-299-8777

13. **International School of Louisiana** isl-edu.org, 1400 Camp St., 504-654-1088

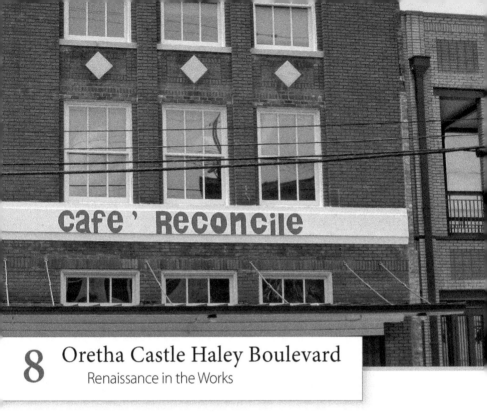

# 8 Oretha Castle Haley Boulevard
## Renaissance in the Works

BOUNDARIES: Oretha Castle Haley Blvd., Erato St., Josephine St., St. Charles Ave.
DISTANCE: 1.39 miles
PARKING: Free parking on the street
PUBLIC TRANSIT: RTA Buses #15 (Freret) and #91 (Jackson-Esplanade), St. Charles Ave. Streetcar

Revival is a theme of many a New Orleans neighborhood, and none may exemplify the concept of comeback more than Oretha Castle Haley Boulevard, one of the main thoroughfares of the historic Central City neighborhood.

A bustling retail strip from the turn of the 20th century through the 1970s, with African American and Jewish merchants running most of the businesses, the street formerly known as Dryades succumbed to disinvestment, poverty, and lack of opportunity. Just blocks away from tony St. Charles Avenue, it became a virtual ghost town, with blighted buildings lining the street and the crime rate continuing to rise.

Fed up with the decline, community activists, civic organizations, and the city of New Orleans embarked on a battle to bring the street affectionately known as O. C. Haley Boulevard—renamed after a beloved civil rights activist in 1989—back to its former glory. It is definitely a work in progress, and much work remains to be done. While some businesses have failed to catch on, there are many signs of success, with restaurants, a cultural center, and a gallery among the businesses that have opened shop.

Since 2006, the O. C. Haley Boulevard Merchants & Business Association has sponsored the Central City Festival, an annual all-day celebration that aims to call attention to the street's rebirth. Over the years, some of the city's hottest local musicians, from Kermit Ruffins to Big Freedia, have performed.

## Walk Description

Begin at St. Charles Avenue and Felicity Street in front of ❶ Houston's Restaurant. Facing Felicity, turn right (northwest) and walk three blocks to O. C. Haley Boulevard. Along this stretch of blocks, you'll pass the Muses Apartments, a mixed-income housing development built after Hurricane Katrina through a variety of public and private partnerships. The complex gets its name from the surrounding streets, which are named for the nine muses of Greek mythology.

Turn right on O. C. Haley. In the first block, at 1712 O. C. Haley, is the ❷ Ashé Cultural Arts Center. Housed in what was once Kaufman's Department Store, it opened in the late 1990s. Its mission: to use art and culture to support community development. In addition to staging an array of performing- and visual-arts shows, the center offers movie screenings, health-and-wellness activities, and outreach programs. The Diaspora Boutique sells an abundance of African merchandise from clothing to jewelry.

Continue walking on O. C. Haley. In the next block, at 1632 O. C. Haley, is the ❸ Friday Night Fights Gym, which stages amateur boxing bouts and typically includes musical and dance performances.

At 1626 O. C. Haley is ❹ YEP Thriftworks, a secondhand store operated by the Youth Empowerment Project, which provides community-based education, mentoring, and employment readiness to underserved youths.

Continue walking to 1504 O. C. Haley, home of the ❺ Southern Food and Beverage Museum, also known as SoFAB. The museum opened in 2008 at Riverwalk Marketplace

## Café Reconcile

If you're looking for flavorful Southern cuisine at an affordable price, look no farther than the corner of Euterpe Street and Oretha Castle Haley Boulevard, home of Café Reconcile. Not only will you leave with a very satisfied tummy, but you'll have contributed to one of New Orleans's greatest nonprofit success stories.

Café Reconcile opened in 2000, the brainchild of the late Rev. Harry Tompson, who joined with other community members in looking for ways to alleviate the violence, substance abuse, and homelessness that were overtaking the neighborhood. They came up with the idea of a restaurant that would train at-risk youth in the city's thriving hospitality industry.

On any given weekday, the place is packed for lunch. Teens age 16 and older, along with young adults up to age 22, work in all areas of the restaurant, from steward to waitstaff to chef. The service is excellent as is the food, with fried catfish, baked macaroni and cheese, and smothered pork chops among the specialties. Since its beginning, Café Reconcile has seen more than 1,500 of its graduates move on to careers in restaurants, hospitals, and other food-service providers.

The café's partners include some of the city's top chefs and restaurateurs, among them Emeril Lagasse and Ralph Brennan. The Emeril Lagasse Foundation Hospitality Center, a special-events space, occupies the second floor.

downtown but outgrew its space. In late 2014, it reopened in this 30,000-square-foot building, the former Dryades Market. In addition to culinary-themed changing exhibits, the museum houses the Museum of the American Cocktail (hey, it's New Orleans); the Leah Chase Louisiana Gallery (named for the legendary New Orleans chef); and the Gallery of the South: States of Taste, where visitors can explore the cooking cultures of other Southern states. Of course, a museum like this wouldn't be complete without food and drink, so an abundance of space is devoted to a cooking-demo kitchen and cooking classes.

New to the boulevard, across from SoFab, is a two-sided historical marker describing the racial violence that took place in the United States between 1877 and 1950. The marker also highlights a four-day period of mass lynchings in 1900, during which White mobs in New Orleans terrorized the city's Black residents, killing at least seven.

In the next block, at the corner of O. C. Haley and Martin Luther King Boulevards, sits the ⑥ New Orleans Jazz Market, a project of the Grammy Award–winning New Orleans Jazz Orchestra, led by drummer Adonis Rose, who also serves as the market's artistic director. The space, once the home of Gator's department store, features a 370-seat theater, a full-service bar, a 500-piece reading library and a digital jazz archive. The market is also home to the New Orleans

Jazz Orchestra School of Music, which offers free music education classes to children on Saturdays and after school.

Walk two blocks to Erato Street, cross O. C. Haley, and turn left to walk on the opposite side of the street. The building at 1307 O. C. Haley is the old Myrtle Banks Elementary School, which opened in 1910 as McDonogh 38 Elementary School but was closed in 2002 because of low enrollment. Six years later, a fire swept through the building, transforming it into a blighted eyesore. As part of the neighborhood's revitalization, Alembic Community Development bought and began renovating the property in 2011. It enjoyed three years of success as the Dryades Public Market, a fresh food emporium, but a dearth of customers forced it to close. As of this writing, its future was unclear.

Walk one block to 1409 O. C. Haley, where you'll be in front of the Harrell Building, a $20 million redevelopment project named for the late Rev. Louis B. Harrell, a longtime resident of Central City and founder of the storefront Living Witness Church of God in Christ in 1981. Harrell was best known for his efforts to improve the quality of life in Central City, starting a clothing-distribution center, a community meal program, a prison ministry, a drug-rehabilitation program, and educational programs aimed at youth. The building houses senior-citizen apartments, office space, and a violence-reduction program called CeaseFire New Orleans. It is also home to the New Orleans Redevelopment Authority, which works with public and private partners to redevelop and revitalize New Orleans neighborhoods like Central City.

As you cross Martin Luther King Boulevard, look to the right at what is called ❼ Hayden Plaza. The plaza is home to a 10-foot bronze sculpture created by artist Frank Hayden to memorialize Dr. King. The sculpture is not an image of King but rather an abstract egg with arms and hands representing the civil rights activist's desire to bring people together. Hayden included a bullet hole in the sculpture to commemorate King's assassination in 1968.

Cross Terpsichore Street. At the corner is Haley's Harvest, one of dozens of community gardens, urban farms, and orchards in underserved New Orleans neighborhoods. In the middle of the block is the ❽ Southern Food and Beverage (SoFAB) Culinary Library and Archive, which boasts an impressive collection of more than 11,000 volumes of cookbooks; more than 5,000 menus; and countless recipes, documents, and other literature about the culinary traditions of the American South. The library is run by the Southern Food and Beverage Museum.

At the end of the block is the neighborhood's crown jewel: ❾ Café Reconcile, a nonprofit restaurant that provides job and life-skills training to at-risk youth (see sidebar on page 45).

Cross Euterpe Street, where at the corner you will see ❿ LOT 1701, an open-air cultural market which offers affordable pop-up spaces to artists, designers, and entrepreneurs with unique wares to sell. The spaces are tiny cottages that have housed everything from a yoga studio to a juice bar.

A block farther is ⓫ **Casa Borrega**, which brought authentic Mexican street food and lively Latino entertainment to the neighborhood when it opened in 2012. The restaurant is housed in an 1891 Greek Revival home that had fallen into disrepair when spouses Hugo Montero and Linda Stone purchased it in 2008. In renovating the building, they used as many existing features as possible while adding materials salvaged from buildings in New Orleans, Texas, and Mexico. The menu boasts such dishes as enchiladas de mole, fish tacos, and huevos rancheros, along with more than 100 tequilas and mezcals.

Walk four blocks to Josephine Street past the headquarters of the Central City Renaissance Alliance, a resident-led community-development organization that envisions a "Central City where the quality of life for everyone is defined by high-quality schools, full employment, an abundance of business and entrepreneurial opportunities, and a healthy and safe environment."

Cross O. C. Haley at Josephine. Turn left on O. C. Haley and continue walking. On your right, the Franz Building (2016 O. C. Haley) houses the Good Work Network, a nonprofit that helps start and grow minority- and women-owned businesses; the Trafigura Work and Learn Center, a youth-employment program comprising several youth-run businesses; and the Southeast Louisiana Women's Business Center.

Walk two blocks and turn right on Felicity Street. At the corner is ⓬ **Café Roma**, which serves up an array of gourmet pizzas, sandwiches, and salads. Walk three blocks back to the starting point on St. Charles Avenue. Along the way, you'll pass ⓭ **The Bank Architectural Antiques** (1824 Felicity), which specializes in antique building materials such as doors, mantels, and period hardware.

*The Southern Food and Beverage Museum celebrates the food and drink of the South through exhibits, tastings, and lectures.*

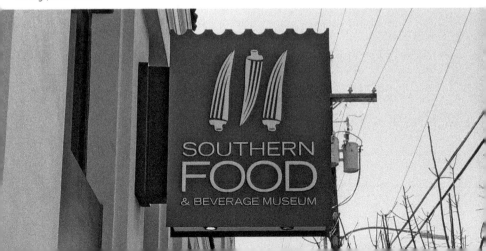

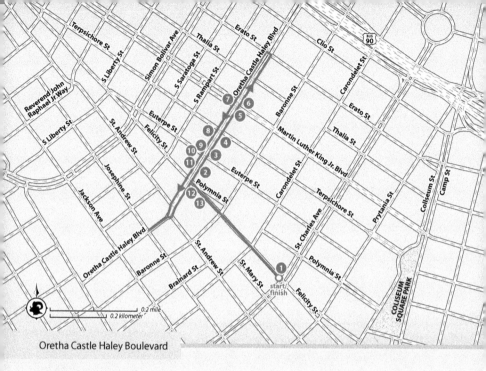

Oretha Castle Haley Boulevard

## Points of Interest

1. Houston's  houstons.com, 1755 St. Charles Ave., 504-524-1578

2. Ashé Cultural Arts Center  ashecac.org, 1712 Oretha Castle Haley Blvd., 504-569-9070

3. Friday Night Fights Gym  1630 Oretha Castle Haley Blvd., 504-522-2707

4. YEP Thriftworks  youthempowermentproject.org/shop-yep, 1626 Oretha Castle Haley Blvd., 504-702-8070

5. Southern Food and Beverage Museum (SoFAB)  sofabinstitute.org, 1504 Oretha Castle Haley Blvd., 504-569-0405

6. New Orleans Jazz Market  thenojo.com/the-market, 1436 Oretha Castle Haley Blvd., 504-371-5849

7. Hayden Plaza (MLK Memorial)  Oretha Castle Haley at Martin Luther King Boulevard

8. Southern Food and Beverage (SoFAB) Culinary Library and Archive  sofabinstitute.org/sofab-culinary-library-and-archive, 1609 Oretha Castle Haley Blvd., 504-569-0405

9. Café Reconcile  cafereconcile.org, 1631 Oretha Castle Haley Blvd., 504-568-1157

10. LOT 1701  lot1701.com, 1701 Oretha Castle Haley Blvd., 504-265-5441

11. Casa Borrega  casaborrega.com, 1719 Oretha Castle Haley Blvd., 504-427-0654

12. Café Roma  caferomauptown.com, 1800 Oretha Castle Haley Blvd., 504-524-2419

13. The Bank Architectural Antiques  thebankantiques.com, 1824 Felicity St., 504-523-2702

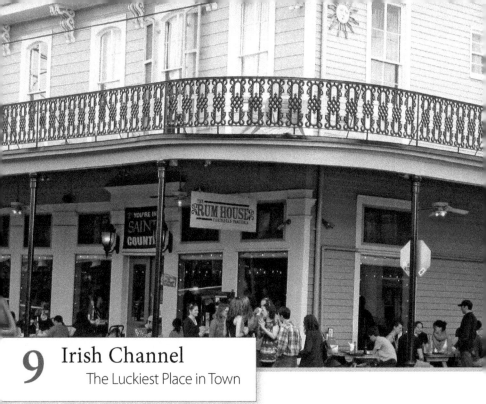

# 9 Irish Channel
## The Luckiest Place in Town

*Above: Sidewalk dining is plentiful along Magazine Street, and the island-inspired Rum House offers some of the best.*

BOUNDARIES: Constance St., Louisiana Ave., Magazine St., Jackson Ave.
DISTANCE: 1.96 miles
PARKING: Free and metered parking on the street; check signs for time limits.
PUBLIC TRANSIT: RTA Bus #11 (Magazine)

Tucked behind the elegant Garden District, the Irish Channel is a largely middle-class neighborhood whose origins date back to the early 19th century. Fearful of the potato famine that was invading their homeland, the Irish settled in the area in droves. It was an easy choice, as many boats ended up along the Mississippi River, dropping passengers off in this very area.

Although the Irish Channel is no longer predominantly Irish, the neighborhood has retained its Irish flair. It boasts some of the liveliest bars in town, including Parasol's and Tracey's. And come March, the Channel is home to the city's biggest and arguably the best St. Patrick's Day celebrations.

Among them is the Irish Channel St. Patrick's Day Club's annual Mass and parade, beginning at St. Mary's Assumption Church before green-clad revelers take to the streets on foot and by float. Parade-goers are strongly encouraged to bring along tote bags—they're likely to head home with more cabbages, potatoes, and beads than they could ever carry in their arms.

But the Irish Channel is more than just shamrocks and leprechauns. The 14-block stretch of Magazine Street between Louisiana Avenue and Jackson Avenue is a haven for shoppers and diners. And if a massage or pedicure is in your plans, there's no shortage of salons and day spas.

## Walk Description

Begin your walk at 2025 Constance St., in front of the old St. Alphonsus Catholic Church, now the ❶ St. Alphonsus Art and Cultural Center. The center is maintained by the Friends of St. Alphonsus, a grassroots organization dedicated to preserving and restoring the 159-year-old church, which served the Irish Catholic community for nearly a century before it was shuttered. The center is open to the public on Tuesdays, Thursdays, and Saturdays from 10 a.m. to 2 p.m. Every March, the group presents "Fun Under the Frescoes," an Irish celebration featuring an array of musical entertainment. St. Alphonsus Parish is now part of St. Mary's Assumption Church, just around the corner on Josephine Street.

Walk two blocks to Jackson Avenue, cross Jackson, and continue walking on Constance, a residential area consisting of restored shotgun and camelback homes. Like so many of the neighborhoods off Magazine Street, this one has experienced a real estate boom over the past several years, its residents enjoying the ease and convenience of nearby restaurants and shops. As you walk down Constance, you may think it's Mardi Gras every day of the week, with many houses sporting decorative parade flags and fences draped with beads. Among the homes you'll pass in the first block is the one-time residence of jazz musician Dominic "Nick" LaRocca at 2218 Constance. LaRocca, a cornetist and bandleader who died in 1961, played for the group that eventually became the Original Dixieland Jazz Band.

Walk four blocks to Third Street. The white dive of a building to the right is ❷ Parasol's, the center of the neighborhood's rollicking St. Patrick's Day festivities. The bar, which opened in 1952, is actually hopping all year long and is especially well known for its succulent roast beef po'boys.

Walk two blocks to Washington Avenue and turn right. Walk another block to Magazine Street, cross Magazine, and turn left. Magazine stretches 6 miles, but the 14 blocks between Jackson and Louisiana Avenues boast some of the coolest, funkiest, most eclectic places in town. As you stroll along Magazine, you'll be mesmerized by the sheer variety, including ❸ Funky Monkey, a secondhand clothing and costume shop; ❹ Fleurty Girl, known for its New Orleans–inspired

T-shirts; and ⑤ Petcetera, a full-service pet boutique offering photography, grooming, and treats like "pupcakes" and "pet me fours." If you like poke, ⑥ Poke Loa, at the corner of Magazine and Louisiana Streets, is a local chain considered one of the best.

At Louisiana, cross Magazine, turn left, and continue walking on the opposite side of Magazine. Over the next 14 blocks, you'll likely be tempted by the many eateries and shops that line the street. Among them are ⑦ Boil Seafood House, where you can get a bucket of spicy-hot boiled crawfish or shrimp; ⑧ Dat Dog, a gourmet hot dog joint; ⑨ Slim Goodies Diner, a popular breakfast spot; ⑩ NOLA Couture, where you can buy New Orleans–themed neckties; ⑪ the Bulldog, an international beer tavern; and ⑫ the Rum House, a Caribbean taqueria.

From the Rum House, at Magazine and Ninth Street, walk another 10 blocks to Jackson Avenue. Along this stretch, you'll pass ⑬ Pippen Lane, an upscale children's clothing and furniture store; ⑭ Sake Café Uptown, where sushi rolls include the Fire Roll, the Po Boy Roll, and the Jazz Roll; and the highly acclaimed ⑮ Coquette, housed in a late 19th-century building that once served as a residence, grocery store, and auto parts store.

During this stretch, you'll also pass through one of Magazine's few residential sections, though many homes have been converted into law offices and other commercial establishments. Amid the homes is ⑯ Tracey's, the neighborhood's other Irish bar. Just a block from Parasol's, Tracey's has an equally yummy roast beef po'boy, along with 20 televisions for patrons to enjoy their favorite local sports teams. Other spots worth stopping at for a bite to eat are ⑰ Molly's Rise and Shine, ⑱ Stein's Deli, and ⑲ District: Donuts Sliders Brew. Any of the flags catch your eye on the route? Stop in at the colorful ⑳ Brad and Dellwen Flag Party, at the corner of Magazine and Jackson, and you may just find a match.

## Points of Interest

① St. Alphonsus Art and Cultural Center  friendsofstalphonsus.org, 2025 Constance St., 504-524-8116

② Parasol's  facebook.com/ParasolsNOLA, 2533 Constance St., 504-302-1543

③ Funky Monkey  www.funkymonkeynola.com, 3127 Magazine St., 504-899-5587

④ Fleurty Girl  www.fleurtygirl.net, 3117 Magazine St., 504-301-2557

⑤ Petcetera  petceteranola.com, 3205 Magazine St., 504-269-8711

⑥ Poke Loa  eatpokeloa.com, 3341 Magazine St., 504-309-9993

*(continued on next page)*

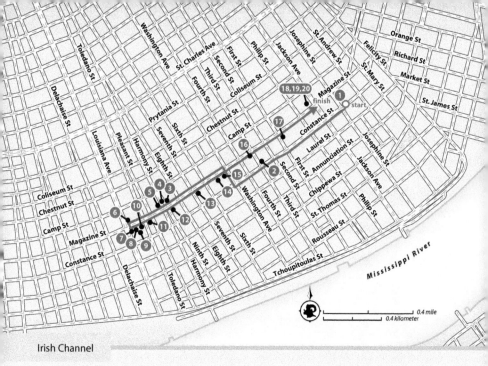

**Irish Channel**

*(continued from previous page)*

- ⑦ Boil Seafood House  boilseafoodhouse.com, 3340 Magazine St., 504-309-4532
- ⑧ Dat Dog  datdognola.com, 3336 Magazine St., 504-324-2226
- ⑨ Slim Goodies Diner  slimgoodiesdiner.com, 3322 Magazine St., 504-891-3447
- ⑩ NOLA Couture  nolacouture.com, 2928 Magazine St., 504-319-5959
- ⑪ The Bulldog  bulldog.draftfreak.com, 3236 Magazine St., 504-891-1516
- ⑫ The Rum House Caribbean Taqueria  therumhouse.com, 3128 Magazine St., 504-941-7560
- ⑬ Pippen Lane  pippenlane.com, 2930 Magazine St., 504-269-0106
- ⑭ Sake Café Uptown  sakecafeonmagazine.com, 2830 Magazine St., 504-894-0033
- ⑮ Coquette  coquettenola.com, 2800 Magazine St., 504-265-0421
- ⑯ Tracey's  traceysnola.com, 2604 Magazine St., 504-897-5413
- ⑰ Molly's Rise and Shine  mollysriseandshine.com, 2368 Magazine St., 504-302-1896
- ⑱ Stein's Market & Deli  steinsdeli.net, 2207 Magazine St., 504-527-0771
- ⑲ District: Donuts Sliders Brew  donutsandsliders.com, 2209 Magazine St., 504-570-6945
- ⑳ Brad and Dellwen Flag Party  2201 Magazine St., 504-527-5211

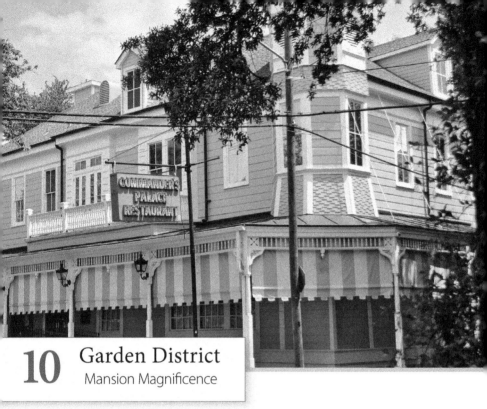

## 10 Garden District
### Mansion Magnificence

---

*Above: In a city filled with fine-dining establishments, Commander's Palace tops the list.*
*photo by Donna Goldenberg*

---

BOUNDARIES: St. Charles Ave., Washington Ave., Coliseum St., Jackson Ave.
DISTANCE: 1.14 miles
PARKING: Free parking on street, but some neighborhood parking is limited to 2 hours.
  Check for signs.
PUBLIC TRANSIT: St. Charles Ave. Streetcar

In a city where elegance and wealth define many a neighborhood, the Garden District may well be the most enviable part of town. It includes a stretch of stately—and busy—St. Charles Avenue, but it is mostly the district's quieter and equally breathtaking interior streets that make it such an appealing place to live, or at least visit.

Listed on the National Register of Historic Places, the Garden District was developed in the early 19th century on what was once the Livaudais Plantation and several other plantations.

# Commander's Palace

From po'boy joints to upscale eateries, New Orleans is a city known for its restaurants. But nothing says "fine dining" quite like Commander's Palace, the Garden District establishment that Emile Commander opened in 1880 to give the neighborhood's well-heeled newcomers an incomparable dining experience.

While many restaurants have come and gone in New Orleans, Commander's, now owned by a branch of the noted Brennan family, continues to draw locals and tourists alike with its award-winning menu of modern Louisiana and Creole fare, from classic turtle soup and crispy pork belly and oysters to griddle-seared Gulf fish and bread-pudding soufflé.

In 2019, *Southern Living* magazine named Commander's the "South's Best Restaurant," and in 2018, *Food & Wine* named it to its "40 Most Important Restaurants of the Past 40 Years." It has also won a bevy of James Beard Foundation Awards. In 2020, sous chef Meg Bickford took over as executive chef, becoming the first woman to helm the legendary kitchen.

Besides dinner, Commander's offers an impressive to-go menu, and if you're celebrating a special occasion, the weekend jazz brunch is as festive as it gets. Before you go, be sure to check commanderspalace .com for the dress code.

Property was sold in parcels to wealthy Americans (specifically, WASPs) who did not want to associate with the Creoles living in the French Quarter.

The Garden District is known for its opulent Greek Revival and Italianate mansions, oak-lined streets, and, of course, magnificent gardens. It's also the neighborhood of choice for such Hollywood celebrities as John Goodman and Sandra Bullock and local luminaries such as former New Orleans Saints quarterback Archie Manning.

Most of the homes remain private residences and are therefore closed to the public. But every year, the Preservation Resource Center, a nonprofit dedicated to preserving the architecture of New Orleans, presents a self-guided holiday tour, giving the curious a chance to see up close the insides of some of the city's most beautiful homes.

# Walk Description

Begin on the south side of St. Charles Avenue at Washington Avenue. Walk one block down Washington to Prytania Street. At the corner to your left is the Rink, a mini shopping mall that includes ❶ **Garden District Book Shop**, one of the city's few remaining independent bookstores; ❷ **Still Perkin'**, a coffeehouse; ❸ **Judy at the Rink**, a gift and home-decor shop; and

④ **Maisonette Shop**, a lux linen store. The mall gets its name from the roller-skating rink that occupied the property for the 1884 World's Fair.

Cross Prytania Street at Washington, turn left, and walk one block to Fourth Street. At the corner, 1448 Fourth, is Colonel Short's Villa, built in 1859 for Col. Robert Henry Short, a cotton merchant. The cast-iron fence surrounding the home features patterns of cornstalks and morning glories; legend has it that Short bought the fence for his wife because she missed her home state of Iowa. The Italianate-style mansion was built by architect Henry Howard, who designed some of Louisiana's most elegant homes, including Nottaway, Louisiana's largest plantation.

Cross Fourth Street and continue walking down Prytania. At 2605 Prytania, at the corner of Third and Prytania, is the Briggs-Staub House, which was built in 1849 and is the only example of Gothic Revival architecture in the Garden District.

Cross Third Street. Across the street, at 2523 Prytania, is the old Our Mother of Perpetual Help, a one-time chapel that best-selling author Anne Rice attended as a child and later bought and converted to a private residence. At more than 13,000 square feet, the house was said to be too small for Rice, who went on to buy and renovate an old orphanage on nearby Napoleon Avenue. Actor Nicolas Cage once owned not only this house but also the LaLaurie House in the Lower French Quarter (see Walk 5), but he lost both to foreclosure.

Continue walking to 2507 Prytania, the Maddox-Mclendon House, a Greek Revival mansion built for Joseph H. Maddox, owner of the *New Orleans Daily Crescent* newspaper, in the 1850s. The interior, which was used in the Jamie Foxx–Leonardo DiCaprio movie *Django Unchained,* features a grand staircase made of mahogany, cypress, and walnut; Baccarat crystal chandeliers; and an opulent ballroom with hand-painted ceilings, among other amenities.

At 2504 Prytania is the ⑤ **New Orleans Women's Opera Guild Home**, which was built in 1859 for Edward A. Davis and donated to the Women's Guild of the New Orleans Opera Association in 1965. The Greek Revival home was designed by noted architect William A. Freret and is open for public tours on Mondays.

Walk one block to 2406 Prytania, the home of French consul general Vincent Sciama. Built in 1905 by attorney John May, the Colonial Revival house was purchased by the Republic of France in 1957 and has housed its consul ever since. According to the Preservation Resource Center, it has undergone numerous renovations over the years but continues to operate as a symbol of the connection and commitment between Louisiana and France.

Cross First Street. The house directly across Prytania is the Bradish Johnson House, a one-time private residence that now serves as the main building for ⑥ **Louise S. McGehee School**, an independent girls' school. The house was designed by James Freret and built in 1872 for wealthy sugar magnate Bradish Johnson. Today, it houses McGehee libraries, classrooms, and the office of the headmistress.

Turn right on First Street. In the middle of the block, at 1420 First St., is the home of former New Orleans Saints quarterback Archie Manning. It is also the childhood home of Manning's three sons, including former NFL quarterbacks Peyton and Eli Manning. An ESPN documentary, *The Book of Manning,* tells the story of growing up Manning and features scenes of father and sons tossing the football in the front yard.

Walk one block to Coliseum Street and turn right. At 2425 Coliseum is the Joseph Merrick Jones House, home of actor John Goodman and the former home of Nine Inch Nails singer Trent Reznor. The house is named for a lawyer who lived there in the mid-1900s. Joseph Merrick Jones also served as secretary for public affairs for the US State Department during World War II and as president of Tulane University.

Walk two blocks to 2627 Coliseum, a Swiss chalet–style mansion built in 1876 by architect William Freret for James Eustis, a US senator and ambassador to France. Today, the house is owned by Academy Award–winning actress Sandra Bullock, whose ties to New Orleans go back to Hurricane Katrina. Following the storm, Bullock adopted the heavily damaged Warren Easton Charter High School in Mid-City and has played a significant role in the school's subsequent success. While in New Orleans, she adopted her son, Louis, and bought the Coliseum Street mansion.

In the next block, at 2707 Coliseum, stands the so-called Benjamin Button House, the primary residence used in the Brad Pitt–Cate Blanchett film *The Curious Case of Benjamin Button*. The Academy Award–winning movie, based on the short story by F. Scott Fitzgerald, was filmed almost entirely in New Orleans. The 8,000-square-foot white center-hall cottage was built in 1832 and has been owned by three generations of the Nolan family. In the movie it served as the old folks' home where Queenie, the resident manager played by Taraji P. Henson, raises Button, who, of course, was played by Pitt.

Continue walking down Coliseum to the corner of Washington Avenue. The mammoth turquoise structure on the right is the legendary ❼ Commander's Palace, a fine-dining institution renowned not just in New Orleans but worldwide. Owned today by Brennan family members Lally Brennan and Ti Adelaide Martin, it dates back to 1880, when Emile Commander opened the only restaurant patronized by the Garden District's distinguished families. Known for its modern Louisiana and Creole cuisine—with Sunday jazz brunch among its most popular meals—Commander's has won countless accolades (see sidebar on page 54).

Cross Washington Avenue and turn right. You're now in front of ❽ Lafayette No. 1 Cemetery, established in 1833 in what used to be known as the city of Lafayette. The cemetery is dedicated to musician Theodore Von LaHache, who founded the New Orleans Philharmonic Society. Among those buried here are Confederate general Harry T. Hayes and Civil War–era Louisiana governor Henry Watkins Allen. Scenes from the movie *Interview with the Vampire* and the CW television series *The Originals* were filmed here. The entrance is a half block down on Washington Avenue. Feel free to stroll through the cemetery—lots of people do—and then return to the entrance.

Walk one block to St. Charles Avenue and turn right. Continue walking to 2618 St. Charles. Known as the Belfort Mansion, this 19th-century Greek Revival home housed seven strangers in the 2000 edition of the MTV reality show *The Real World: New Orleans*. (The series filmed again in New Orleans in 2010, this time housing its cast on Dufossat Street in Uptown.)

Walk another block to 2524 St. Charles to the Greek Revival home known as the Claiborne Cottage. Anne Rice lived here as a teenager, and the home is the setting for her book *Violin*.

Continue walking to 2220 St. Charles. The ❾ **House of Broel** was built in the 1850s by George Washington Squires. The house, which today is used as a wedding and party venue, features the Mystic Ballroom, a lavish setting with ornate chandeliers and original black-marble fireplaces. The house is open for public tours.

Walk to the corner of St. Charles and Jackson Avenue. Your tour ends here.

*Mausoleums line the rows at Lafayette No. 1 Cemetery.    photo by Shutterstock/Christian Ouellet*

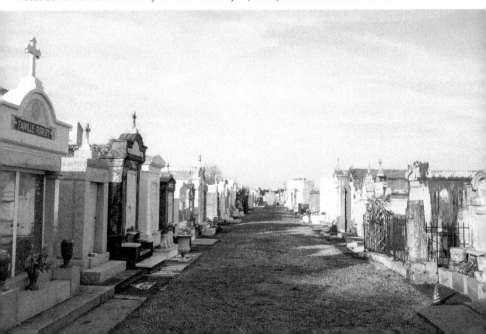

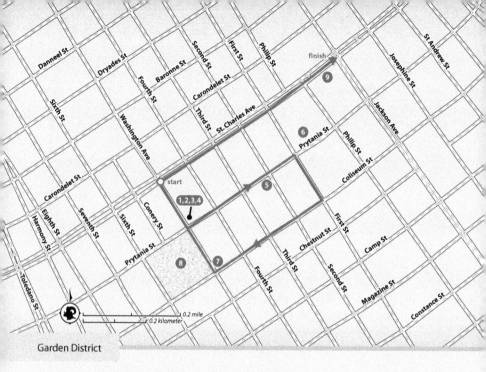

Garden District

## Points of Interest

1. Garden District Book Shop  gardendistrictbookshop.com, 2727 Prytania St., 504-895-2266

2. Still Perkin'  2727 Prytania St., 504-899-0335

3. Judy at the Rink  facebook.com/judyattherink, 2727 Prytania St., 504-891-7018

4. Maisonette Shop  maisonetteshop.com, 2727 Prytania St., 504-437-1850

5. New Orleans Women's Opera Guild Home  neworleansopera.org/category/womens-guild, 2504 Prytania St., 504-899-1945

6. Louise S. McGehee School  mcgeheeschool.com, 2343 Prytania St., 504-561-1224

7. Commander's Palace  commanderspalace.com, 1403 Washington Ave., 504-899-8221

8. Lafayette No. 1 Cemetery  nola.gov/cemeteries, 1400 Washington Ave., 504-658-3781

9. House of Broel  houseofbroel.com, 2220 St. Charles Ave., 504-522-2220

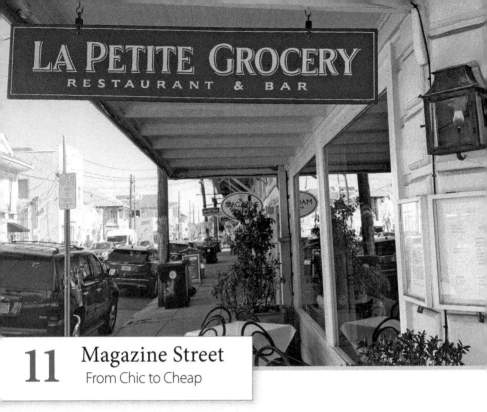

## 11 Magazine Street
### From Chic to Cheap

Above: La Petite Grocery is the award-winning restaurant of Chef Justin Devillier.

BOUNDARIES: Magazine St., Louisiana Ave., State St.
DISTANCE: 2 miles
PARKING: Metered parking on Magazine; free in the neighborhood, but check signs for time limits.
PUBLIC TRANSIT: RTA Bus #11 (Magazine). For $3 you can buy a Jazzy Pass, which lets you take unlimited bus rides in a single day.

In a city brimming with cool streets, from funky Frenchmen Street in Faubourg Marigny to ritzy Royal Street in the French Quarter, none may be cooler than Magazine Street, a 6-mile stretch that runs from Audubon Park to the Central Business District.

Magazine has it all, from high-end boutiques to secondhand stores, from po'boy joints to fine-dining bistros, and from sports bars to music clubs. There are yoga studios, art galleries, and antiques stores, not to mention day spas, coffeehouses, and dessert cafés.

Three Mardi Gras parades—Muses, Nyx, and Thoth—roll on portions of Magazine, as does the Irish Channel St. Patrick's Day Parade. Other events on Magazine include Art for Arts' Sake, a gallery-hopping affair signaling the start of the fall arts season. The annual Champagne Stroll, held the Saturday evening before Mother's Day, gives last-minute shoppers a chance to buy the perfect gift for Mom.

Magazine follows the length of the Mississippi River crescent and takes in such neighborhoods as Uptown, the Garden District, the Irish Channel, the Warehouse District, and Downtown. Because Magazine is also included in our Lower Garden District and Irish Channel tours (Walks 7 and 9, respectively), this walk is limited to the stretch between State Street and Louisiana Avenue in Uptown.

## Walk Description

Begin at the corner of State and Magazine, in front of ❶ Reginelli's, a popular New Orleans pizza chain, and across the street from ❷ Picnic Provisions & Whiskey, which boasts a picnic-style menu of fried chicken, Cajun potato salad, and brownie s'mores, among other offerings. In the first couple of blocks, you'll pass several other restaurants, including the upscale-yet-casual ❸ Avo and ❹ Bistro Daisy, housed in a quaint yellow cottage. Avo specializes in Italian cuisine; Bistro Daisy serves French food with a Southern twist.

Cross Nashville Avenue and continue down Magazine. To your left, at the corner of Nashville and Magazine, is ❺ Saba, an Israeli restaurant, whose chef, Alon Shaya, has been nominated five times for James Beard Awards. If you're in the market for a New Orleans T-shirt, check out ❻ Dirty Coast (5631 Magazine). You won't find X-rated T-shirts here—for those, you'll have to head to Bourbon Street. What you will find are some of the cleverest, most New Orleans–centric shirts in town. Examples include "That Voodoo You Do," "There Is a House in New Orleans" (in reference to Saints and the Superdome), and "Union, Justice, Crawfish."

The mammoth building to your right is ❼ Whole Foods Market, which when it was being developed in 2001 met with a mix of reactions, from euphoria to rage. Opponents argued the store would be too big for the neighborhood; supporters liked the idea of developing a blighted but historic building, the old Arabella bus barn. Today, it's hard to imagine this block without Whole Foods, where if you're lucky you might just see New Orleans Saints quarterback Drew Brees—who lives nearby—pushing a cart. And with so many movies being filmed in New Orleans these days, celebrity sightings aren't uncommon: Will Ferrell, Emma Roberts, and Sarah Jessica Parker have shopped here, and Whole Foods was also one of the stomping grounds of the *Top Chef: New Orleans* cast.

The next block, between Joseph Street and Octavia Street, is chock-full of unique and fun shops. Among them are ⑧ Swap, a consignment store billed as a "haven for fashionable and budget-conscious women"; ⑨ Hazelnut, a home-decor store co-owned by local celebrity and former *Mad Men* actor Bryan Batt; and ⑩ EarthSavers, known for its luxurious spa treatments.

Although not on the route, ⑪ Octavia Books (513 Octavia St.) is worth the detour if you're a book lover. Turn right on Octavia and walk two blocks. Octavia Books is one of the city's few independent bookshops and is stocked with genres of all kinds. The shop hosts book clubs, author signings, children's programs, and more.

Cross Jefferson at ⑫ CC's Coffee House, part of a chain of local coffee shops. To your right is Poydras Home, a nursing home and assisted-living center founded in 1817 as a home for women and children left widowed and orphaned by the yellow fever epidemic. Named for businessman and philanthropist Julien Poydras (see Walk 3), it moved to its present site on Magazine in 1857. The next stretch of blocks is largely residential, though you will pass a handful of businesses, such as ⑬ Guy's Po-Boys, where you can get a roast beef topped with fries and cheddar cheese (we kid you not).

At 5116 Magazine, between Soniat and Dufossat Streets, is St. Katharine Drexel Preparatory School, a Catholic girls' school that until the 2013–14 academic year had been the century-old Xavier Preparatory School, run by the Sisters of the Blessed Sacrament. Because of financial issues, the sisters announced they were closing after 98 years of educating primarily African American girls. Determined to keep the school open, a group of Xavier Prep alumni purchased the campus and led the way for its transformation to St. Katharine Drexel Prep.

At the corner of Soniat and Magazine is ⑭ Henry's Uptown Bar, a century-old institution that, according to legend, was a favorite watering hole of JFK assassin Lee Harvey Oswald, who was born and raised in New Orleans. In its coverage of the 50th anniversary of JFK's assassination, *The Times-Picayune* wrote extensively about Oswald's time in New Orleans, including the story of him being thrown out of Henry's when the owner refused to turn on the television coverage of his arrest for passing out "Hands Off Cuba" pamphlets on Canal Street.

In the next block is ⑮ Tito's Ceviche and Pisco, one of the few Peruvian eateries in town. As the name suggests, Tito's has an impressive menu of ceviche as well as pisco-based cocktails. Pisco is a type of brandy produced in Peru and Chile. A block from Tito's is ⑯ Pizza Domenica, the casual offshoot of Domenica in the Roosevelt Hotel downtown (see Walk 2, Canal Street).

For breakfast or lunch, check out ⑰ Surrey's Uptown. The place is generally packed, but the wait for such dishes as huevos rancheros, crabmeat omelets, or fried green tomatoes is worth it. Just next door, at the corner of Bordeaux Street and Magazine, is ⑱ Le Bon Temps Roule, another classic Uptown bar. *Laissez les bons temps rouler* means "Let the good times roll," and this live-music venue lives up to its name, serving free oysters on Fridays and $1 beers during Saints games. The Soul Rebels, a New Orleans brass band, performs on Thursday nights.

Other restaurants scattered over the next several blocks include ⓳ **Apolline**, an upscale Southern bistro where you can have a drink custom-made to suit your mood and taste; ⓴ **La Boulangerie**, a French pastry shop; and ㉑ **Del Fuego Taqueria**, where you can people watch while sipping a margarita from the patio.

Several boutiques can be found on this stretch as well, including ㉒ **The Bead Shop**, which carries an amazing inventory of beads and beading supplies and has a stringing room where you can make your own necklace, bracelet, or earrings. If you're a beginner, one of the store's beading experts will walk you through the process.

Walk to the corner of Magazine and Napoleon. To the right, facing Napoleon, is the ㉓ **Carol Robinson Gallery**, which operates out of a restored 19th-century house. It features the works of such artists as Mississippi painters Jere Allen and Robert Malone, sculptor Ron Dale, Japanese painter Masahiro Arai, local pastel artist Sandra Burshell, and abstract painter Karen Jacobs. Also on display are three-dimensional works, including Roddy Capers's blown-glass vases and Michael Yankowski's wooden altarpieces.

Cross Napoleon Avenue and continue walking down Magazine. To your right is ㉔ **Ms. Mae's**, a 24-hour dive known for cheap drinks and convenient restrooms during Carnival parades. To the left is Lawrence Square, where at almost any time of the day you'll see a rousing game of basketball; and the Second District headquarters of the New Orleans Police Department. Next to the police station is St. George's, an independent Episcopal school founded in 1969.

Across Magazine and next to Ms. Mae's is the legendary oyster house ㉕ **Casamento's**, established in 1919 by Italian immigrant Joe Casamento. The place is known as much for its tile decor as it is for its fried-oyster loaves. If you're in the market for a tutu or tiara, stop in at ㉖ **Uptown Costume Shop**, which also stocks a bounty of masks, wigs, and feather boas, not to mention Elvis apparel.

Walk one block to the corner of Magazine and General Pershing Street. To the right is the highly rated ㉗ **La Petite Grocery**, whose owner and executive chef, Justin Devillier, was a contestant on Bravo TV's *Top Chef: New Orleans*. The building once housed a full-service grocery store with a barn in the back to house delivery carriages. Devillier, who's won much acclaim for his culinary creativity (can you say blue-crab beignets?), has been named a James Beard Award finalist multiple times.

Walk two blocks to the corner of Marengo Street, where you'll see Neal Auction Company to the right. Established in 1983, it holds auctions six times a year, with each comprising fine art and antiques from estates, private collections, and cultural institutions. During the next stretch, you'll pass several high-end clothing boutiques, including the Uptown shop of New Orleans jewelry designer 28 **Mignon Faget**, at the corner of Magazine and Peniston.

Yet another award-winning restaurant, the French- and Italian-inspired 29 **Lilette**, has sat at the corner of Magazine and Antonine since 2000. Housed in a one-time apothecary, Lilette was once dubbed "the sexiest dining room in New Orleans" by *Travel & Leisure* magazine. Owner and chef John Harris has been named a James Beard finalist for Best Chef: South, and *Food & Wine* named him one of the best new chefs in America.

In the next block, at 3606 Magazine St., is the home of WRBH, the city's radio station for the blind and visually impaired. The station's mission is "to turn the written word into the spoken word so that the blind and print handicapped receive the same ease of access to current information as their sighted peers." WRBH is the only full-time reading service on the FM dial in the United States, and one of only three in the world. Because of the station's streaming capability, it reaches people worldwide.

Walk three blocks to Louisiana Avenue past 30 **Mahoney's Po-Boys and Seafood**, which was once featured on the hit Food Network show *Diners, Drive-Ins and Dives*. Mahoney's boasts a long list of po'boys, but its signature sandwich is the Peace Maker, a po'boy stuffed with fried oysters, bacon, and cheddar cheese.

At Louisiana, catch RTA Bus #11 for your trip back to the starting point. Of course, if you're up to it, feel free to walk beyond Louisiana before making the trek back.

*Casamento's has been serving oysters and other seafood delights for over a century.*

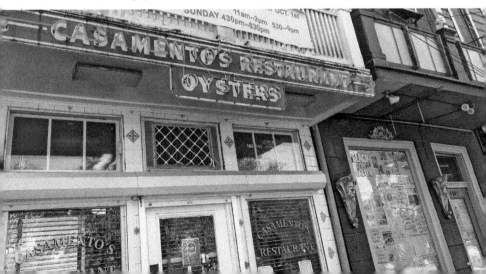

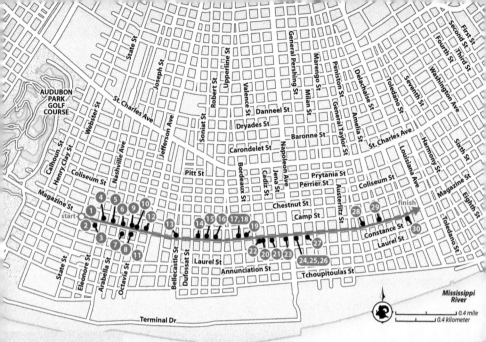

Magazine Street

## Points of Interest

1. Reginelli's Pizzeria  reginellis.com, 5961 Magazine St., 504-899-1414

2. Picnic Provisions & Whiskey  nolapicnic.com, 741 State St., 504-266-2810

3. Avo  restaurantavo.com, 5908 Magazine St., 504-509-6550

4. Bistro Daisy  bistrodaisy.com, 5831 Magazine St., 504-899-6987

5. Saba  eatwithsaba.com, 5757 Magazine St., 504-324-7770

6. Dirty Coast  dirtycoast.com, 5631 Magazine St., 504-324-3745

7. Whole Foods Market–Arabella Station  wholefoodsmarket.com/stores/arabellastation, 5600 Magazine St., 504-899-9119

8. Swap  swapboutique.com, 5530 Magazine St., 504-324-8143

9. Hazelnut  hazelnutneworleans.com, 5515 Magazine St., 504-891-2424

10. EarthSavers  earthsaversonline.com, 5501 Magazine St., 504-899-8555

11. Octavia Books  octaviabooks.com, 513 Octavia St., 504-899-7323

12. CC's Coffee House  ccscoffee.com, 900 Jefferson Ave., 504-891-4969

13. Guy's Po-Boys  facebook.com/guyspoboysnola, 5259 Magazine St., 504-891-5025

14. Henry's Uptown Bar  facebook.com/henrys.uptown.bar, 5101 Magazine St., 504-324-8140

15. Tito's Ceviche and Pisco  titoscevichepisco.com, 5015 Magazine St., 504-267-7612

16. Pizza Domenica  pizzadomenica.com, 4933 Magazine St., 504-301-4978

17. Surrey's Uptown  surreysnola.com, 4807 Magazine St., 504-895-5757

18. Le Bon Temps Roule  lbtrnola.com, 4801 Magazine St., 504-895-8117

19. Apolline  apollinerestaurant.com, 4729 Magazine St., 504-894-8869

20. La Boulangerie  laboulangerienola.com, 4600 Magazine St., 504-269-3777

21. Del Fuego Taqueria  delfuegotaqueria.com, 4518 Magazine St., 504-309-5797

22. The Bead Shop  beadshopneworleans.com, 4612 Magazine St., 504-895-6161

23. Carol Robinson Gallery  carolrobinsongallery.com, 840 Napoleon Ave., 504-895-6130

24. Ms. Mae's  facebook.com/msmaesNOLA, 4336 Magazine St., 504-218-8035

25. Casamento's  casamentosrestaurant.com, 4330 Magazine St., 504-895-9761

26. Uptown Costume Shop  facebook.com/uptowncostumeanddancewear, 4326 Magazine St., 504-895-7969

27. La Petite Grocery  lapetitegrocery.com, 4238 Magazine St., 504-891-3377

28. Mignon Faget  mignonfaget.com, 3801 Magazine St., 504-891-2005

29. Lilette  liletterestaurant.com, 3637 Magazine St., 504-895-1636

30. Mahony's Po-Boys and Seafood  mahonyspoboys.com, 3454 Magazine St., 504-899-3374

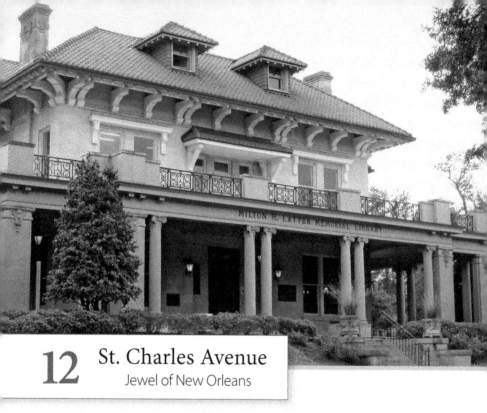

# 12 St. Charles Avenue
## Jewel of New Orleans

*Above: The Milton H. Latter Memorial Library was once the residence of department store magnate Mark Isaacs and later lumber mogul Frank B. Williams.*

BOUNDARIES: St. Charles Ave., Louisiana Ave., Eleonore St.
DISTANCE: 2.77 miles
PARKING: Free on St. Charles and in the surrounding neighborhood, but bear in mind that parking on some residential streets is limited to 2 hours.
PUBLIC TRANSIT: St. Charles Avenue Streetcar

If there's one street in New Orleans that's made for walking, it's magnificent St. Charles Avenue, the so-called Jewel of America's Grand Avenues and one of the top 10 thoroughfares in the United States as ranked by the American Planning Association in 2007.

Stretching 6.4 miles from the Central Business District to Riverbend, St. Charles Avenue is known for its exquisite mansions, many of which date back to the mid-19th century, when it became home to New Orleans's wealthiest and most powerful citizens.

Most of the mansions still stand today, though some have been converted to luxury apartment buildings, bed-and-breakfasts, or, in one case, a public library. Numerous churches, synagogues, schools, and businesses, along with Tulane and Loyola Universities and Audubon Park, also make their homes on the grand, oak-lined avenue.

The best way to see St. Charles Avenue is on foot or by streetcar, so the following walking tour allows for both. Take your time as you marvel at the avenue's beauty, then hop on the streetcar, grab a window seat, and enjoy the view once again.

# Walk Description

Begin at 5809 St. Charles, in front of the Colonial Revival mansion known as the Wedding Cake House because of its many layers and adornments. Probably the most photographed house on the avenue, it dates back to the late 19th century, when it served as the home of Nicholas Burke, a wholesale grocer. The house has undergone numerous renovations and was rebuilt in 1907 after an electrical fire.

Walk one block, cross Nashville Avenue, and check out the George Palmer House at 5705 St. Charles. Though not nearly as large as most of the mansions on the avenue, the plantation-style house is famous for being built to resemble Tara, the O'Hara family home in *Gone with the Wind*. Another historic house once stood at this site; it was built for Lawrence Fabacher, who founded Jax Brewery (see Walk 6).

Walk two blocks to the Benjamin-Monroe Mansion at 5531 St. Charles. The 22-room Italianate Beaux Arts Renaissance Revival house was designed by noted New Orleans architect Emile Weil for businessman Emmanuel V. Benjamin in 1912. It was later owned by J. Edgar Monroe, a shipbuilder and philanthropist, followed by several other owners. Next to the Benjamin-Monroe house is ❶ Danneel Playspot, one of the city's nearly 120 parks and playgrounds.

Walk one block and cross Jefferson Avenue. To the right is the ❷ Jewish Community Center, which has occupied the corner of St. Charles and Jefferson since 1948. The JCC actually dates back to 1855 with the formation of the Young Men's Hebrew and Literary Society. The society eventually became the Young Men's Hebrew Association and later the Young Men's and Young Women's Hebrew Association. It changed its name to the Jewish Community Center upon moving to its current location, the site of the former Jewish Children's Home. The JCC offers an array of programming, from summer camp and nursery school to health-and-wellness activities and Jewish holiday celebrations.

Next to the JCC, at 5300 St. Charles, is De La Salle High School, home of the Cavaliers, which was founded as a Catholic school for boys in 1949 but which became coed in 1992. De La Salle

# Latter Library

With its lavish grounds and neo-Italianate design, the mansion between Dufossat and Soniat streets fits in perfectly with the other palatial homes along St. Charles Ave. But instead of housing people, it houses books.

Listed on the National Register of Historic Places, the Milton H. Latter Memorial Library was built in the early 20th century as the private residence of Mark Isaacs, founder of Maison Blanche, one of the city's legendary department stores.

When Isaacs died in 1912, lumber magnate Frank B. Williams bought the house. His son Harry Williams, an aviation pioneer, was married to Marguerite Clark, an American stage and silent-film actress. The couple inherited the house after the elder Williams's death and lived there until 1936, when Harry Williams died in a plane crash. Clark lived there for another three years before moving to New York.

Racetrack owner Robert Eddy bought the house in 1937, and a decade later, he sold it to real estate executive Harry Latter. Looking for a way to memorialize their only son, Milton, who was killed in World War II, Latter and his wife immediately donated it to the city for use as a public library.

Although the library has undergone numerous renovations over the years, it has preserved many of the formal rooms as reading rooms, along with some of the home's original adornments, among them Czechoslovakian chandeliers, Dutch murals, and South American mahogany paneling.

Regular events at Latter include book sales, film screenings, author visits, summer reading programs, early-literacy events, and adult programming. The library is open seven days a week, so be sure to stop in for a visit while walking the avenue. Call 504-596-2625 or visit nolalibrary.org for hours.

is part of the Brothers of the Christian Schools network, which has 1,500 schools in 85 countries.

Walk one block to Dufossat Street. To the right is the ③ **Milton H. Latter Memorial Library**, a former private home that is undoubtedly the most stunning of the New Orleans Public Library's 14 branches (see sidebar above).

Walk one block to 5010 St. Charles. The Tudor-style house was built in 1909 for Joseph Vaccaro, founder of the Standard Fruit and Steamship Company, one of the first businesses to import bananas from Honduras to New Orleans. Standard Fruit eventually became the Dole Food Company.

To the left, at 5005 St. Charles, is the home of the Orleans Club, an exclusive women's club. Built in 1868 as a wedding gift from Colonel William Lewis Wynn to his only daughter, Ann Elizabeth Wynn Garner, the house remained in private hands until 1925, when a group of 300 women purchased it for a club dedicated to women's interests and the arts. Today, members host a variety of cultural-arts programs along with debutante teas and other society functions.

Walk three blocks to 4717 St. Charles. The Richardsonian Romanesque Revival mansion is easily one of the largest houses on the avenue, at 22,000 square feet and four stories. It was built over three years in the early 20th century by cotton magnate W. P. Brown, founder of Hibernia Bank, as a wedding gift for his wife. In 2011, two floors of the house were open to the public for the first time as part of a tour to benefit the New Orleans Museum of Art.

Walk one block to St. George's Episcopal Church (4600 St. Charles), which got its start as a diocesan mission just before the Civil War at the corner of Berlin (now General Pershing Street) and Magazine Streets. The present-day church was dedicated in 1900, its architecture and stained-glass windows among its most noted features. In 1969, church leaders opened St. George's Episcopal School on nearby Camp Street. One of the school buildings is located on the site of the original mission. Among other programs, the church hosts the Dragon Café, which serves free breakfast every Sunday morning to the hungry and poor.

Walk another block to 4534 St. Charles. The stone Mediterranean-style villa was built in 1906 for William Mason Smith, president of the New Orleans Cotton Exchange. To the left, at 4521 St. Charles, is the ❹ Academy of the Sacred Heart, a Catholic girls' school that is part of a network of Sacred Heart schools around the world. Sacred Heart dates back to the early 19th century, when it was based in the French Quarter. In 1847 it moved to a Greek Revival mansion on St. Charles, to accommodate the growing number of families who were moving Uptown. When that building proved to be too small, a new Colonial Revival–style structure went up in its place in 1900. Over the years, the school has undergone numerous renovations and expansions—so many, in fact, that the only remnant of its origins is a wrought-iron fountain topped with a swan.

Continue walking down St. Charles and cross at Napoleon Avenue. During Carnival season, this intersection is one of the most popular places for parade-watching, with dozens of parades making the turn onto St. Charles from Napoleon. One thing you're sure to notice as you continue down St. Charles are all the beads hanging from the trees, the result of float riders missing their targets on the streets. On Fat Tuesday, as well as the days leading up to it, the streets are wall-to-wall people, especially for such parades as Bacchus, Orpheus, Muses, and Rex.

The restaurants at or near this intersection attract their share of crowds as well, during Carnival and throughout the year. They include ❺ Superior Seafood, which offers a full-service oyster bar and spectacular views of the St. Charles streetcar line; ❻ Fat Harry's, a legendary watering hole; and ❼ New Orleans Hamburger & Seafood Company, part of a local chain of casual eateries where you can also get beignets.

From St. Charles and Napoleon, walk a block to 4238 St. Charles, home of ❽ Touro Synagogue, the sixth-oldest synagogue in the country and the first outside the 13 original colonies.

On the first Friday of the New Orleans Jazz & Heritage Festival, Touro, a Reform synagogue, sponsors Jazz Fest Shabbat, a rousing Sabbath service featuring some of the city's top musicians along with the temple's choir and cantor.

New to the neighborhood is ❾ The Chloe, a 14-room hotel housed in a 19th-century mansion. The hotel features a pool, patio, and bar along with a restaurant led by Chef Todd Pulsenelli, who is known for contemporary Creole fare.

Walk three blocks to ❿ The Columns, a boutique hotel in a late-19th-century Italianate house designed by Thomas Sully, considered one of New Orleans's greatest architects. Listed on the National Register of Historic Places, The Columns was once the home of cigar magnate Simon Hernsheim. Featuring a grand mahogany staircase and many other original details, it later became a boardinghouse, and, in 1953, a hotel. If time allows, stop in for a drink in the Victorian Lounge, once the main dining room, or enjoy a bite to eat on the grand veranda. Several movies and TV shows have been shot here, including Brooke Shields's 1978 film debut, *Pretty Baby,* and the popular FX anthology series *American Horror Story: Coven.*

As you continue walking down St. Charles, you'll pass numerous luxury condo developments. At 3636 St. Charles is ⓫ Superior Grill, a Mexican restaurant known for its happy hours and for being a popular gathering spot for Mardi Gras parades. The best seats in the house are on the patio, where you can watch the streetcars roll by over a plate of crawfish enchiladas and a frozen margarita. Equally fun but with a different vibe is ⓬ The Delachaise, a wine bar at 3442 St. Charles. The outdoor patio, with its twinkling lights, is the perfect spot to share a bottle of wine and a cheese plate.

The walk officially ends at St. Charles and Louisiana Avenue, but feel free to continue the stroll—until your feet give out—and catch the streetcar back to the starting point. The St. Charles Ave. Streetcar was recently named a National Historic Landmark and is well worth the experience.

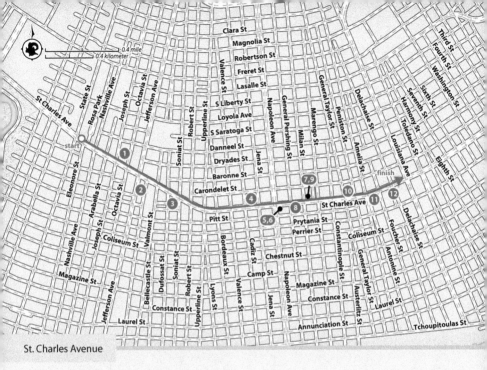

St. Charles Avenue

## Points of Interest

1. Danneel Playspot  5501 St. Charles Ave. at Octavia Street

2. Jewish Community Center  nojcc.org, 5342 St. Charles Ave., 504-897-0143

3. Milton H. Latter Memorial Library  nolalibrary.org, 5120 St. Charles Ave., 504-596-2625

4. Academy of the Sacred Heart  ashrosary.org, 4521 St. Charles Ave., 504-891-1943

5. Superior Seafood  superiorseafoodnola.com, 4338 St. Charles Ave., 504-293-3474

6. Fat Harry's  fatharrysnola.com, 4330 St. Charles Ave., 504-895-9582

7. New Orleans Hamburger & Seafood Company  nohsc.com, 4141 St. Charles Ave., 504-247-9753

8. Touro Synagogue  tourosynagogue.com, 4238 St. Charles Ave., 504-895-4843

9. The Chloe  thechloenola.com, 4125 St. Charles Ave., 504-313-6807

10. The Columns  thecolumns.com, 3811 St. Charles Ave., 504-899-9308

11. Superior Grill  superiorgrill.com, 3636 St. Charles Ave., 504-899-4200

12. The Delachaise  thedelachaise.com, 3442 St. Charles Ave., 504-895-0858

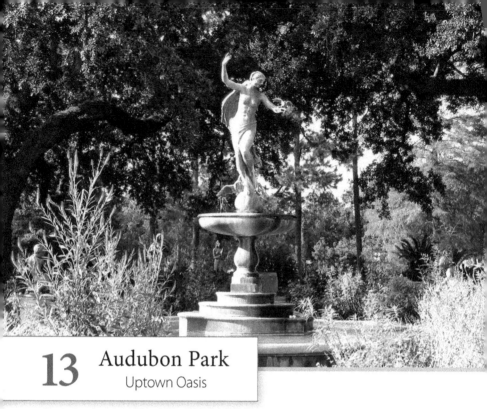

# 13 Audubon Park
## Uptown Oasis

*Above: The Gumbel Memorial Fountain, at the entrance of the park, is the work of Austrian sculptor Isidore Konti.*

BOUNDARIES: St. Charles Ave., Exposition Blvd., Mississippi River, Walnut
DISTANCE: 1.8 miles–3.2 miles (two options)
PARKING: Free parking along St. Charles Ave.; 2-hour parking in neighborhood
PUBLIC TRANSIT: St. Charles Ave. Streetcar

The folks at the Audubon Nature Institute call Audubon Park an "urban oasis," and they couldn't have come up with a more appropriate description. With its duck-filled lagoon, ancient live oaks, and serene sitting areas, Audubon offers a respite to anyone looking to escape the pressures of life.

In historic Uptown New Orleans across from Tulane University, Audubon Park has a rich and fascinating history, having once been home to Native Americans and, many years later, the nation's first commercial sugarcane plantation. During the Civil War, the site alternately hosted a Confederate camp and a Union hospital.

The city acquired the land in 1871 for the purpose of hosting The World's Industrial and Cotton Centennial Exposition of 1884, Louisiana's first world's fair. At the time, the park was called Upper City Park, but city planners renamed it Audubon Park in 1886 in honor of artist-naturalist John James Audubon, who painted many of his iconic *Birds of America* in Louisiana.

With its development handed over to landscape architect John Charles Olmsted—whose family's firm designed New York's Central Park—Audubon became a full-fledged city park. Today, the 300-acre recreational area includes a 1.8-mile jogging trail, a 2.2-mile dirt path, a golf course, riding stables, picnic shelters, playgrounds, tennis courts, and soccer fields.

Local celebrities such as New Orleans Saints quarterback Drew Brees, who lives in the neighborhood, are regular visitors to Audubon Park. And with the city's exploding film industry, other stars—Harrison Ford and Woody Harrelson among them—have been known to partake of the park's amenities.

## Walk Description

Begin at the front entrance of ❶ Audubon Park, on St. Charles Ave. across from Tulane University. Spend some time in the circular garden. Its fountains, sculpture, and vast array of blooms make this one of the park's most enticing stops.

Continue onto the paved jogging trail in front of *The Travelers,* three sculptures by artist Deborah Masters. The trail is divided into a section for bikers and another for walkers and joggers. Be sure to stay on the correct side, and if you bring your dog, remember that leashes are mandatory.

Turn right (west) at the sculptures and begin walking along the park's duck-filled lagoon. You're likely to see ducks, swans, and geese meandering along the shore, their honks and quacks mingling with the rumble of St. Charles Avenue streetcars. Visitors are welcome to bring stale bread to feed to them.

Continue walking west along the trail. Even on the most sweltering of days, Audubon's ancient live oak trees provide enough shade to make walking bearable. Take some time to marvel at these spectacular moss-draped wonders of nature—they make Audubon so special.

As you circle the trail and head south, you'll see the mansions of Walnut Street to your right and Cecile's Crepe Myrtle Grove to your left. One of many wedding venues in the park, the grove features gazebos at each end, a circular path, an open field, and dozens of crepe myrtle trees, whose pink and red blooms are at their peak in the summer. The area was dedicated to Cecile Usdin, a park patron who considered this her favorite spot on the park grounds.

To the right is the Walnut Street Playground, built with a generous donation from Drew Brees and his wife, Brittany. The playground promotes interactive physical, cognitive, visual, and hearing experiences for all children and provides an especially welcoming environment for children with mobility challenges. Playground features include wheelchair-accessible areas; a bongo drum panel that encourages children to have fun with rhythm; a Braille and clock panel; and a "ZipKrooz," a two-way ride similar to a zip line that includes a track with a bucket seat for children with limited core strength. The playground also offers traditional attractions, such as slides, parallel bars, a balance beam, and a tightrope bridge.

As you continue walking south, you'll notice the ❷ Audubon Golf Course, an 18-hole golf course that features contoured Bermuda fairways, manicured Tif-Eagle greens, four lagoons, and exquisite landscaping. Entry is limited to those who are playing, but the ❸ Audubon Clubhouse Café, inside the clubhouse, is open to the public. Grab a table on the wraparound veranda and enjoy the view.

As you approach Magazine Street, you may take one of two routes—continuing around the jogging trail or crossing Magazine Street and heading to the Riverview. This will add 1.4 miles to the walk but will take you right up to the banks of the Mississippi River.

If you prefer to stay on the trail, continue walking on the trail past the rear entrance of the park; if you want to check out the Riverview, cross Magazine at West Drive. Note that Magazine is a heavily traveled roadway, so be extra careful as you make your way across. Continue walking south. The buildings to your right are luxury condominiums. To your left is the award-winning ❹ Audubon Zoo, which, like the park itself, is part of the Audubon Nature Institute's conglomeration of nature attractions. With its vast array of exotic animals, the zoo is well worth a separate visit.

Around the 1-mile point, you'll have to cross a railroad track to get to the south side of the park. The Riverview is commonly known as ❺ The Fly, a reference to a butterfly-shaped river-viewing shelter built in the 1960s and demolished in the 1980s. The area is an ideal spot for picnicking, kite-flying, Frisbee-tossing, or relaxing with a good book. Benches line the riverfront, giving visitors an up-close view of barges and ships traveling to and from the Port of New Orleans.

Make your way around the Fly, past the soccer and baseball fields, and turn north onto Exposition Boulevard, which will take you to the southeast corner of the park, past the tennis courts. Exposition eventually turns into East Drive, where one of the first sites you'll see on the left (near Annunciation Street) is the magnificent Tree of Life, one of the park's oldest trees and another popular wedding venue. Although no signs identify the tree, its massive roots and limbs, many of which droop to the ground, make it difficult to miss. Stop at the tree and take in its beauty before continuing down the roadway to the Labyrinth, a meditative space with a formal entry arch, walking trail, and benches. Adjacent to the Labyrinth are the ❻ Cascade Stables, a state-of-the-art riding facility that offers lessons, show training, and 2-mile guided rides around the park.

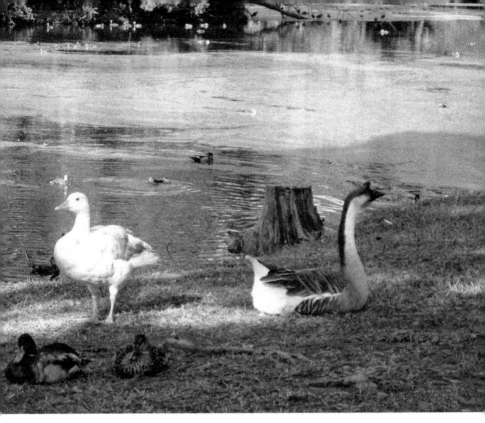

*Ducks, swans, and other birds are common sights in and along Audubon Park's lagoons.*

Cross Magazine Street and return to the north side of the park. Get back on the jogging trail and continue walking north. On the left, you'll see the Newman Bandstand, the only location in the park where amplified music is allowed. In that same area is the Louisiana Roll of Honor, a World War I memorial.

Continue walking north past the stately homes of Exposition Boulevard to your right and—about halfway between Magazine and St. Charles—you'll see Bird Island, which has been part of Audubon Park for more than a century. The natural bird habitat is home to egrets, herons, and other wading birds.

Continue walking north toward St. Charles Avenue. As you get closer, you'll see the tower of the Holy Name of Jesus Church and hear the rumbling of streetcars. Turn northwest and return to the front entryway.

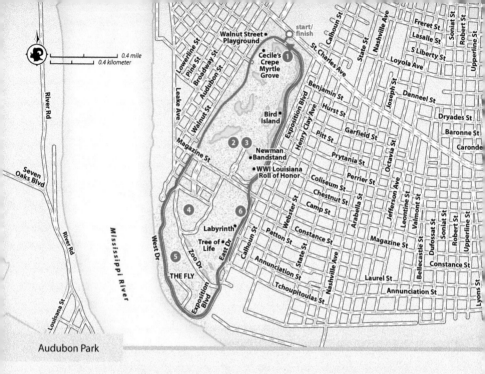

Audubon Park

## Points of Interest

1. Audubon Park  audubonnatureinstitute.org, 6500 Magazine St., 504-581-4629

2. Audubon Golf Course  audubonnatureinstitute.org/golf, 6500 Magazine St., 504-212-5290

3. Audubon Clubhouse Café  audubonnatureinstitute.org/clubhouse-cafe, 6500 Magazine St., 504-212-5282

4. Audubon Zoo  audubonnatureinstitute.org/zoo, 6500 Magazine St., 504-861-2537

5. The Fly  audubonnatureinstitute.org/explore-audubon-park/riverview, 504-861-2537

6. Cascade Stables  cascadestables.net, 504-891-2246

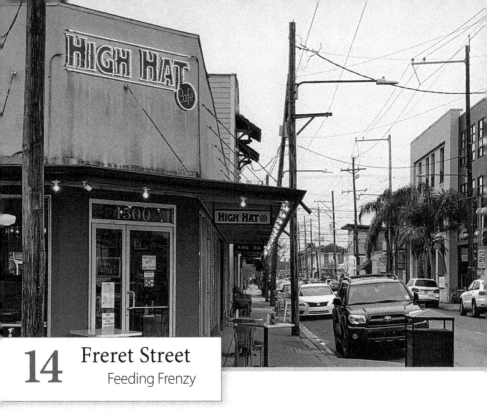

# 14 Freret Street
## Feeding Frenzy

*Above: High Hat Cafe is known for its Southern cuisine, especially Louisiana catfish.*

BOUNDARIES: Freret St., Jefferson Ave., Napoleon Ave.
DISTANCE: 1.04 miles
PARKING: Free lot at Freret and Jena Sts., free street parking
PUBLIC TRANSIT: RTA Bus #15 (Freret)

It's no secret that New Orleans is one of the world's preeminent dining destinations, with some of the finest restaurants to be found in the French Quarter, the Warehouse District, and along Magazine Street. Now you can add Freret Street, between Jefferson and Napoleon Avenues, to the culinary mix.

Freret Street, named after the 19th-century mayor William Freret, is a haven for foodies. You won't find any fine-dining eateries on this eight-block stretch, but what you will discover are places specializing in fun and creative fare—gourmet hot dogs, for instance, and craft cocktails, along with gelato, kolaches, and even a Louisiana take on the Philly cheesesteak. The growing number of businesses is equally impressive: salons, a comic book store, an art gallery, a garden center, a kickboxing studio, and a clothing boutique, among others.

The transformation of Freret from nearly dead to alive and kicking is nothing short of a miracle. Though the street had been a thriving commercial strip in the mid-20th century, suburban sprawl and the murder of Bill Long, a beloved Freret Street baker, in the 1980s left the strip decayed and depressed.

Enter the Freret Business and Property Owners Association, a group of citizens who vowed "to establish an image that Freret Street is a safe, vibrant, easily accessible destination to shop, dine, play, work, and live." They succeeded beyond anyone's imagination, and the growth of Freret continues to this day, with even more restaurants and businesses in the works.

## Walk Description

Begin your walk at the corner of Napoleon Avenue and Freret Street in front of the building that once housed Holy Rosary Academy and High School, a Catholic school that closed in 2019 because of declining enrollment. Across the street is a parking lot that is transformed into the Freret Market on the first Saturday of every month (except July and August). The market features art and produce vendors, live music, a children's area, and restaurants serving up their specialties.

Walk one block to Jena Street. A little advice before you continue: Make sure you're hungry, and unless you know exactly where you want to dine, snack, or drink (maybe all three), browse a few menus so you have a feel for the variety of fare being served. Of course, nothing says you can't try something at every stop, right?

On the corner of Jena and Freret is ❶ High Hat Cafe, located in the building that once housed Bill Long's Bakery and Deli. High Hat is known for its Southern cuisine, and among its specialties are fried catfish, barbecue shrimp, pimento cheese, and heavenly sides like pimento mac and cheese, stone-ground grits, and braised greens. Next door, ❷ Ancora is known for its Neapolitan pizza.

❸ Acropolis, at 4510 Freret, is one of the few Greek restaurants in New Orleans, specializing in such fare as gyros, moussaka, and souvlaki. If you go, don't miss the six-onion soup, a creamy blend of six onions topped with puffed pastry. Just next door to Acropolis are ❹ the Rook Cafe, a coffeehouse geared to tabletop-gaming fans, and ❺ Sarita's Grill, a Latin-fusion café and one of the first businesses to open on the so-called New Freret.

Cross Cadiz Street and you'll be in front of ❻ The Company Burger, one of the first of a proliferation of gourmet burger restaurants to open in New Orleans over the past five years. Among

# Cure

Neal Bodenheimer, a mixologist, was among the first proprietors to take his chances on Freret Street in 2009, and his decision to open the craft-cocktail bar Cure in an old firehouse inspired other businesses to follow suit.

Today, Freret is a thriving culinary corridor, with Cure one of its most popular destinations. Since opening, Cure has been named to *Esquire*'s list of Best Bars in America, *Travel & Leisure*'s list of America's Best Cocktail Bars, and *Food & Wine*'s Best Cocktail Bars in the US.

It's easy to see why. The menu features a fascinating collection of libations, including a brandy-based drink called My Ride is Here and a Cognac creation called Cock N' Bull. Beer and wine selections are equally impressive.

"This classy bar has perfected the delicate act behind the perfectly balanced cocktail," *Travel & Leisure* wrote of Cure. "With a tremendous selection of spirits, a variety of house-made bitters, and a talented crew with a freakish bent for creativity, cocktails here never disappoint."

No need to starve at Cure either. The menu includes a variety of cheese trays and small plates, such as smoked trout dip, white bean hummus, and goat cheesecake.

its accolades are inclusion in *Food & Wine*'s "Best Burgers in America" and CNN's "Top 10 Burgers in America." Its specialty is simple: twin patties, two slices of American cheese, house-made bread-and-butter pickles, and red onions.

Continue walking down Freret to Valence Street, where you'll pass one of the newest eateries on the block, ❼ Val's. Housed in an old Conoco gas station, Val's offers an array of gourmet tacos, from crispy beef belly to green molé chicken.

Cross Valence Street, where at the corner is ❽ Mojo Coffee House, a Wi-Fi café offering breakfast and lunch. In the middle of the block is ❾ Humble Bagel. Bagel shops have come and gone in New Orleans, but Humble Bagel seems to be filling a demand for the real deal, with kettle-boiled bagels like those found in America's best bagel shops.

Cross Upperline Street. In this block, you'll find ❿ Gasa Gasa (Japanese for "easily distracted"), a music venue that boasts a regular lineup of local bands and performers, along with art exhibitions, film screenings, and recording sessions.

Cross Robert Street and continue walking past yet another place for tacos, ⓫ Mr. Tequila Bar and Grill. At the end of the block, enjoy the colorful, funky scene that is ⓬ Dat Dog, a hot dog joint that began in a 465-square-foot shed before moving to bigger digs—an old service station—across the street. That was in 2011, and the place continues to grow in popularity with a second location on Magazine Street and a third on Frenchmen Street in the Marigny. Named to Zagat's "Top 10 List of Franks Worth Traveling For," Dat Dog offers such dogs as alligator sausage, spicy chipotle veggie, and turducken (a trio of duck, turkey, and chicken). Even the fries are worth the splurge, especially the White Trash Fries, topped with chili, sour cream, guacamole, onions, cheese, and jalapenos.

Continue down Freret past two more restaurants—⑬ Mint, a Vietnamese bistro and bar, and ⑭ Origami Sushi (because what's a culinary corridor without sushi?). Walk two more blocks and cross Freret at Jefferson Avenue, the halfway point of the Freret food crawl.

Beginning at ⑮ Starbucks, walk two blocks to the 5000 block of Freret, a stretch that includes ⑯ Liberty Cheesesteaks, which serves up authentic Philly cheesesteaks (with onions and Cheez Whiz); a dive called ⑰ the Other Bar; ⑱ Iacovone Kitchen, a gourmet take-out spot; ⑲ Good Bird, a rotisserie chicken joint; ⑳ City Greens, offering an array of salads and power bowls; and ㉑ Blaze Pizza, known for its custom-built artisan pies.

Cross Robert Street. At the end of the block is ㉒ Cure, the craft-cocktail bar whose owners get much of the credit for the Freret Street revival (see sidebar on page 79).

As you make your way back to Napoleon, you'll pass several more restaurants: ㉓ Midway Pizza, known for its deep-dish pie; ㉔ The Kolache Kitchen, home of the traditional Czech pastry (savory and sweet); and ㉕ Piccola Gelateria, which serves 18 flavors of gelato and sorbetto. Just off Jena Street is ㉖ Bearcat Cafe, a popular all-day breakfast spot.

## Points of Interest

① High Hat Cafe  highhatcafe.com, 4500 Freret St., 504-754-1336

② Ancora Pizzeria & Salumeria  ancorapizza.com, 4508 Freret, 504-324-1636

③ Acropolis  acropolisonfreret.com, 4510 Freret, 504-309-0069

④ The Rook Cafe  facebook.com/therookcafe, 4516 Freret St., 618-520-9843

⑤ Sarita's Grill  4520 Freret St., 504-324-3562

⑥ The Company Burger  thecompanyburger.com, 4600 Freret St., 504-267-0320

⑦ Vals  valsnola.com, 4632 Freret St., 504-356-0006

⑧ Mojo Coffee House  facebook.com/mojofreret, 4700 Freret St., 504-875-2243

⑨ Humble Bagel  humblebagel.com, 4716 Freret St., 504-355-3535

⑩ Gasa Gasa  gasagasa.com, 4920 Freret St., 504-338-3567

⑪ Mr. Tequila Bar and Grill  mrtequilanola.com, 5018 Freret St., 504-766-9660

⑫ Dat Dog  datdog.com, 5030 Freret St., 504-899-6883

⑬ Mint Modern Bistro & Bar  mintmodernbistro.com, 5100 Freret St., 504-218-5534

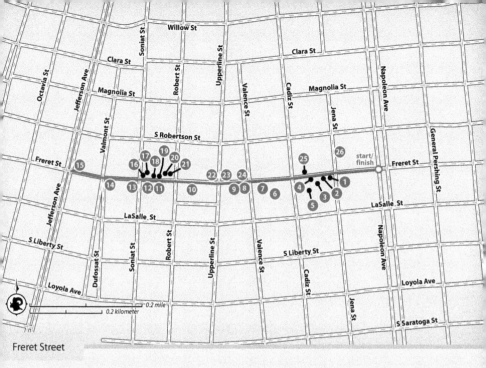

Freret Street

14. Origami Sushi  origaminola.com, 5130 Freret St., 504-899-6532

15. Starbucks  5335 Freret St., 504-861-1302

16. Liberty Cheesesteaks  libertycheesesteaks.com, 5041 Freret St., 504-875-4447

17. The Other Bar  5039 Freret St., 504-460-6414

18. Iacovone Kitchen  iacovonekitchen.com, 5033 Freret St., 504-516-2307

19. Good Bird  goodbirdnola.com, 5031 Freret St., 504-875-4447

20. City Greens  eatcitygreens.com, 5001B Freret St., 504-323-2893

21. Blaze Pizza  blazepizza.com, 5001 Freret St., 504-603-3085

22. Cure  curenola.com, 4905 Freret St., 504-302-2357

23. Midway Pizza  midwaypizzanola.com, 4725 Freret St., 504-322-2815

24. The Kolache Kitchen  thekolachekitchen.com, 4701 Freret St., 504-218-5341

25. Piccola Gelateria  piccolagelateria.com, 4525 Freret St., 504-493-5999

26. Bearcat Cafe  bearcatcafe.com, 2521 Jena St., 504-309-9011

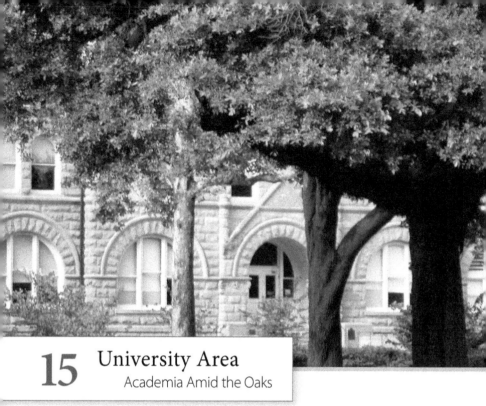

## 15 University Area
### Academia Amid the Oaks

*Above: Gibson Hall is the main administrative building at Tulane University and one of the oldest buildings on campus.*

BOUNDARIES: St. Charles Ave., Calhoun St., Willow St., Broadway St.
DISTANCE: 2.3 miles
PARKING: Free parking on St. Charles, free 2-hour residential parking in neighborhood
PUBLIC TRANSIT: St. Charles Ave. Streetcar

New Orleans is home to myriad colleges and universities, but none is as stunning as the campuses of Tulane and Loyola Universities, which front historic St. Charles Avenue across from Audubon Park in a neighborhood of stately, jaw-dropping mansions.

Chartered in 1912, Loyola University New Orleans is one of 28 Jesuit colleges and universities in the United States. Spread out over 24 acres, it boasts an 11:1 student ratio and five colleges: business, humanities and natural sciences, law, music and fine arts, and social sciences.

Tulane, one of the nation's preeminent research universities, was founded as the Medical College of Louisiana in 1834, eventually merging with the public University of Louisiana. It debuted as the private Tulane University in 1884 when benefactor Paul Tulane, a wealthy merchant, donated more than $1 million in land, cash, and securities "for the promotion and encouragement of intellectual, moral, and industrial education." Tulane's academic divisions include architecture, social work, business, science and engineering, medicine, law, liberal arts, and public health and tropical medicine. In the fall of 2014, Tulane unveiled its newest gem: Yulman Stadium, bringing Green Wave football back to campus after a 40-year absence.

Tulane and Loyola enjoy a harmonious relationship. The two schools host many joint programs, and students with meal plans can dine at either campus.

## Walk Description

Start at the north corner of St. Charles at Calhoun Street. ❶ Loyola's Communications/Music Complex is to the right. The 115,000-square-foot structure is one of Loyola's newer, more modern buildings. It houses the College of Music and Fine Arts, the School of Mass Communication, and the Louis J. Roussel Performance Hall, Loyola's largest performance venue.

Continue down St. Charles Avenue past Marquette Hall, the oldest building on campus. Listed on the National Register of Historic Places, Marquette houses the office of Loyola's president as well as other administrative offices.

Next to Marquette is the iconic ❷ Holy Name of Jesus Church, one of the city's most spectacular Catholic churches and home to such Loyola events as baccalaureate ceremonies, choral concerts, and school-year-opening Mass. The church was founded in 1886. Stained glass with various memorials adorns the upper windows.

Cross West Road and continue down St. Charles past Gibson Hall, ❸ Tulane's main administrative building. The oldest building on Tulane's Uptown campus, Gibson was built in 1894 in the Richardsonian Romanesque style of stone over brick. It houses the admissions office and the offices of the university president, provost, and other senior-level executives. The TULANE UNIVERSITY sign in front of Gibson is one of the most photographed spots on campus.

Turn right onto campus just before Law Road. The building to the left is Tilton Hall, home to the Amistad Research Center, a manuscripts library for the study of ethnic history and culture and race relations in the United States. Built in 1902, the building also houses the Murphy Institute of Political Economy, which supports research in public policy, public affairs, and civic engagement and seeks to educate students on the most challenging of economic, moral, and political problems.

Turn right between Tilton and Dinwiddie Halls, past the rear side of Gibson. At the center stairway of Gibson, turn left and walk through the Academic Quad. As you walk through the Quad, marvel at the spectacular live oak trees and, if it's springtime, garden upon garden of hot-pink azaleas. Tulane has been named to BuzzFeed's list of 41 Scenic College Campuses That Were Made for Instagram, and its lushness and architecturally historic buildings are certainly two reasons why.

To the right is the Richardson Memorial Building, which houses Tulane's acclaimed School of Architecture. Along the path, look for the Mardi Gras bead sculpture titled *Bead Three,* where strands of colorful plastic beads hang like moss. The 21-foot steel-and-acrylic "trees" replaced the famous Bead Tree, which was removed from campus in 2019 because of extensive termite and lightning damage. Just as they did with the real tree, students enjoy gathering at *Bead Three* to add to its decor.

As you walk through the quad, keep an eye out for several pieces of outdoor sculpture. Among them are *Timber,* a structure made of glass, steel, and wood by Gene Koss, and *Arcs in Disorder,* one of the trademark works of French artist Bernar Venet.

Continue walking down the middle walkway past Cudd Hall and Mussafer Hall to the left and Stanley Thomas Hall to the right. You are now in Tulane's science and engineering hub, where in addition to the traditional sciences, students can choose from such majors as biomedical engineering, evolutionary biology, and computer science. The Donna and Paul Flower Hall for Research and Innovation is a contemporary four-story building set behind a towering oak. With its cutting-edge labs, Flower serves as a vital part of the city's growing bioscience and chemical-engineering sectors.

Just ahead is ❹ PJ's Coffee, where you can stop for an iced latte, mocha, or lemonade—that is, unless students are between classes. That's when the café is at its busiest, with professors and students grabbing cups of joe en route to their next class.

Cross Freret Street, one of the major streets that runs through campus, and continue straight onto McAlister Place, a landscaped pedestrian mall and popular gathering spot. In the fall of 2013, actors Channing Tatum and Jonah Hill filmed parts of *22 Jump Street* along the walkway, attracting hundreds of giddy, photo-snapping students—all on their way to class.

To the right is Devlin Fieldhouse, home of Tulane's men's and women's basketball teams. Just past Devlin is the ❺ Lavin-Bernick Center for University Life, also known as the LBC. The LBC is home to a ❻ Barnes & Noble bookstore, dining venues, conference rooms, study lounges, and outdoor patios, including one that overlooks the LBC quad. On Friday afternoons, students begin the weekend with "Fridays on the Quad," a party featuring bands, food trucks, inflatables, and other activities.

Across from the LBC is the ultramodern Goldring/Woldenberg Business Complex, home of the A. B. Freeman School of Business. Next door is McAlister Auditorium, which boasts the world's largest self-suspended concrete dome. The auditorium is used for concerts, lectures, and the occasional movie set. One such movie was the political comedy-drama *Our Brand Is Crisis,* produced by George Clooney and starring Sandra Bullock.

Turn left in front of the LBC and walk a block to Newcomb Place. At the corner is the Commons, a modern, 77,000-square-foot building that houses a state-of-the art dining facility on two levels. When dinner service ends at 10 p.m., the dining room becomes a late-night study space.

Cross Newcomb and enter the Newcomb Quad, once the home of H. Sophie Newcomb Memorial College, the first women's coordinate college within a US university. Walk around the quad, beginning with Dixon Hall to your left. Dixon is one of the city's most popular performance venues and home to the acclaimed Summer Lyric Theatre. Other buildings on this part of campus include Newcomb Hall, the architectural centerpiece of Newcomb College; Dixon Hall Annex, where the New Orleans Shakespeare Festival at Tulane and other performance ensembles are based; and Woldenberg Art Center, home to the ❼ Newcomb Art Museum, which is free and open to the public. The museum regularly presents original exhibitions that explore socially engaged art, civic dialogue, and community transformation.

Circle around the quad and turn left at Newcomb Place. Walk a block past the Caroline Richardson Building and the University Health Center to Willow Street. Turn left on Willow and walk two blocks to Broadway Street. Though not part of Tulane's campus, Broadway is the center of Greek life at Tulane, with many of the homes occupied by fraternities and sororities.

Walk one block to Zimple Street. The high-rise to your left is the Barbara Greenbaum House at Newcomb Lawn. Continue down Broadway past a strip of commercial establishments, including ❽ Crêpes à la Cart and ❾ Mushroom New Orleans, which sells used and out-of-print CDs, posters, and other music-related merchandise.

The large yellow building at the corner of Broadway and Burthe is home to Tulane Hillel, which serves Tulane's significant Jewish student community. ❿ Rimon at Hillel's Kitchen, under the direction of chef Dan Esses, is a fully kosher restaurant open to the public, with menu items such as matzah ball soup, falafel, and bagels.

Continue walking south on Broadway toward St. Charles Avenue. ⓫ Campus Connection, at the corner of Maple Street, stocks an array of Greek merchandise as well as a wide variety of Tulane T-shirts, sweatshirts, and hats.

At St. Charles, turn left and walk to Audubon Place, one of the Crescent City's most exclusive neighborhoods. Audubon Place is private, so you'll only be able to catch a glimpse from outside the gates. Do take note of #2 Audubon Place, the white-pillared mansion that fronts St. Charles. Built in 1907, the Georgian Revival house was the home of United Fruit Company magnate Samuel Zemurray for decades before he donated it to Tulane to serve as the official residence of the university president.

Cross Audubon Place and continue walking past Gibson Hall back the starting point.

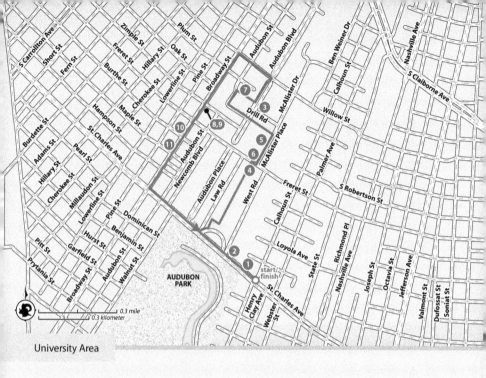

University Area

## Points of Interest

1. Loyola University New Orleans  loyno.edu, 6363 St. Charles Ave., 504-865-3240
2. Holy Name of Jesus Church  hnjchurch.org, 6367 St. Charles Ave., 504-865-7430
3. Tulane University  tulane.edu, 6823 St. Charles Ave., 504-865-5000
4. PJ's Coffee  pjscoffee.com, 7001 Freret St., 504-865-5705
5. Lavin-Bernick Center  lbc.tulane.edu, McAlister Place, 504-865-5190
6. Barnes & Noble  tulane.bncollege.com, McAlister Place, 504-865-5913
7. Newcomb Art Museum  newcombartmuseum.tulane.edu, Newcomb Quad, 504-865-5328
8. Crêpes à la Cart  crepesalacartnola.com, 1039 Broadway St., 504-866-2362
9. Mushroom New Orleans  themushroomnola.com, 1037 Broadway St., 504-866-6065
10. Rimon at Hillel's Kitchen  rimontulanehillel.com, 912 Broadway St., 504-909-9919
11. Campus Connection  campusconnection.cc, 800 Broadway St., 504-866-8552

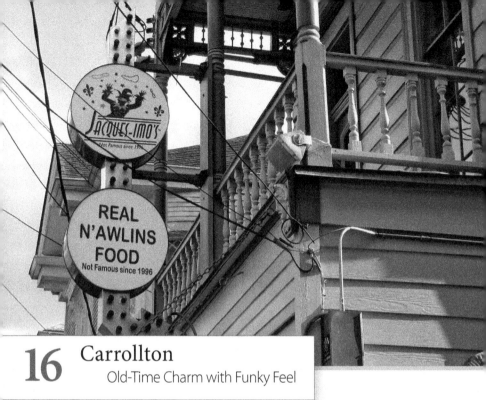

# 16 Carrollton
## Old-Time Charm with Funky Feel

Above: Fried grits, potato-crusted drum, and stuffed quail are among the tempting menu items at Jacques-Imo's.

BOUNDARIES: St. Charles Ave., S. Carrollton Ave., Oak St., Dublin St.
DISTANCE: 1.54 miles
PARKING: Free parking on St. Charles, metered parking on Carrollton
PUBLIC TRANSIT: St. Charles Ave. Streetcar

The Carrollton neighborhood has a rich and fascinating history dating back to the mid-18th century, when, as the town of Carrollton, it was the seat of Jefferson Parish. Carrollton was annexed by New Orleans in 1874, but remnants of the old days remain—including the pillared structure that once housed the town's courthouse but which has been home to several schools ever since.

With its majestic oak trees, streetcar line, and quaint commercial districts, the neighborhood still has a small-town feel. Yet in spite of its many transformations over the years, it is one of the city's most vibrant neighborhoods. Much of the credit goes to the revitalization of Oak Street, a funky street with old-time charm, where you'll find galleries, restaurants, cafés, secondhand stores, and more.

These days, Oak Street is synonymous with po'boys, the ubiquitous sandwich that's as popular in New Orleans as cheesesteaks are in Philly. You won't find any famous po'boy shops on Oak, but every November, the street shuts down for the Oak Street Po-Boy Festival. With more than 30 vendors serving such po'boys as shrimp and crabmeat, barbecued oyster, drunken pig, and brisket with blue cheese, dieting—or maybe even fasting—the week before is highly advisable!

# Walk Description

Begin at the corner of St. Charles Avenue and South Carrollton Avenue in front of ❶ Cooter Brown's, a popular dive sports bar with an impressive oyster bar and beer selection. Cross St. Charles, but be extra-careful, as this is one of the area's busiest intersections.

Continue two blocks on Carrollton to the stretch between Hampson and Maple Streets. Dating back to the 1850s, the building to your right once served as the courthouse for the town of Carrollton. It has also been home to several schools, including John McDonogh No. 23 School, Benjamin Franklin High School, and Lusher Extension School. Audubon Charter School vacated the building in May 2014. Plans to convert the building into an assisted-living facility are being considered.

Cross Maple Street. Though not included on this walk, Maple Street is certainly worth a side visit. Its boutiques, restaurants, cafés, and bars are especially popular with students from nearby Tulane and Loyola Universities.

Continue down Carrollton past the Wilkinson-Bruno House, a Gothic Revival–style home built in 1846 and listed on the National Register of Historic Places. Adjacent to this house, between Oak and Zimple Streets, is St. Andrew's Episcopal Church. Cross Oak, turn left, cross Carrollton, and continue walking on the north side of Oak, in front of an old bank building that now houses a nail salon and ❷ Pho Bistreaux, a Vietnamese restaurant.

Oak Street is like a small town unto itself where you can get your hair cut, your bike fixed, your pet groomed, or your arm tattooed. Oak extends all the way to the river, but this walk will take you five blocks to Joliet Street. Along the north side are ❸ Truburger, serving gourmet burgers and hot dogs; ❹ Haase's, a children's shoe and clothing store that has been in business for decades; and ❺ Eclectic Home, an interiors shop.

Cross Oak at Joliet and continue along the south side of Oak. The two most popular venues on Oak—❻ Jacques-Imo's and the ❼ Maple Leaf Bar—are situated side by side between Cambronne and Dante Streets. Do yourself a favor and plan a night around these two landmarks.

Jacques-Imo's is a casual eatery that serves some of the tastiest food in town, from shrimp-and-alligator-sausage cheesecake to blackened redfish topped with crab chili hollandaise. On any given night, the place is packed, and reservations are accepted only for parties of five or more. If you want a real dining adventure, consider reserving the colorful pickup truck that's parked in front. In the back of the truck is a table for two, the perfect spot for people-watching.

The Maple Leaf Bar is one of the city's most venerable music clubs, offering an array of music from jazz and blues to zydeco and funk. Among the club's regulars are the Rebirth Brass Band, funk and R&B musician Jon Cleary, and Bonerama. Over the years, unannounced sit-in guests have included the likes of Bruce Springsteen and Bonnie Raitt.

Next door to the Maple Leaf Bar is ⑧ Frenchy Gallery, whose owner, Frenchy, travels the country painting scenes from live performances such as sporting events and music festivals.

Walk four blocks back to Carrollton Avenue, past even more restaurants, galleries, and shops. They include ⑨ Glue Clothing Exchange, a vintage garment store; ⑩ Live Oak Café, a popular breakfast spot; ⑪ Blue Cypress Books, a secondhand book shop; and ⑫ Oak Wine Bar, which also has live music. Grab a cup of java at ⑬ Rue de la Course at the corner of Carrollton and Oak, which, like Pho Bistreaux across the street, is housed in an old bank building.

Turn right at Carrollton and walk four blocks to Maple Street. Turn right at Maple in front of ⑭ Madigan's Bar and continue walking in the heart of the Riverbend neighborhood. The strip shopping center on the left features one of the best sandwich-and-shake shops in town: ⑮ The Milk Bar, where you can order such concoctions as Psycho Chicken, Cattle Fodder, and Wolf Me Down. Shakes include Mocha Madness, Butterscotch Hop, and Strawberry Fields.

Cross Dublin Street, turn left, and walk a block to Hampson Street. In this neighborhood, you'll find almost every ethnic food imaginable—Mexican at ⑯ La Mansion, Spanish at ⑰ Barcelona Tapas, and Japanese at ⑱ Hana, among the choices. At the corner of Hampson and Dublin is ⑲ Yvonne LaFleur, an upscale boutique known for its custom millinery, signature fragrances, and resplendent ball and wedding gowns. Also on Hampson is ⑳ Sno-la Snowballs, known for its cheesecake-stuffed snowballs.

Turn right at Carrollton and continue walking past ㉑ Camellia Grill, perhaps the most famous landmark in the whole neighborhood. The Grill, as locals call it, opened in 1946, and—except for a few years post-Katrina—has been serving up burgers, omelets, waffles, and other diner fare ever since. The food is good, but the waiters are better: they're funny, friendly, and full of spunk.

Continue down Carrollton past the Shell service station, cross St. Charles Avenue, and return to the starting point—unless you want one last refreshment at ㉒ New Orleans Original Daiquiris, to your right at 8100 St. Charles. Remember: in New Orleans, you can take your drinks to go.

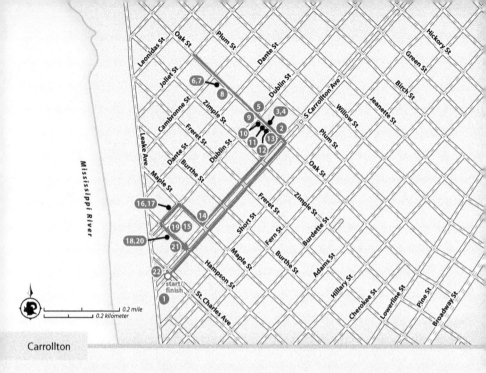

Carrollton

## Points of Interest

1. Cooter Brown's  cooterbrowns.com, 509 S. Carrollton Ave., 504-866-9104

2. Pho Bistreaux  orderphobistreaux.com, 1200 S. Carrollton Ave., 504-304-8334

3. Truburger  8115 Oak St., 504-218-5416

4. Haase's  haases.com, 8119 Oak St., 504-866-9944

5. Eclectic Home  eclectichome.net, 8211 Oak St., 504-866-6654

6. Jacques-Imo's  jacques-imos.com, 8324 Oak St., 504-861-0886

7. Maple Leaf Bar  mapleleafbar.com, 8316 Oak St., 504-866-9359

8. Frenchy Gallery  frenchylive.com, 8319 Oak St., 504-861-7595

9. Glue Clothing Exchange  glueneworleans.com, 8206 Oak St., 504-782-0619

10. Live Oak Café  liveoakcafenola.com, 8140 Oak St., 504-265-0050

11. Blue Cypress Books  bluecypressbooks.com, 8126 Oak St., 504-352-0096

12. Oak Wine Bar  oaknola.com, 8118 Oak St., 504-302-1485

*Camellia Grill opened in 1946 and has been serving classic diner fare ever since.*

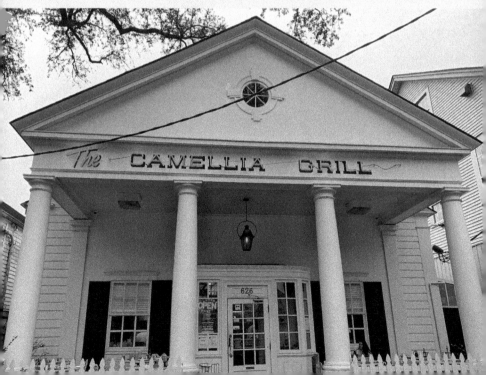

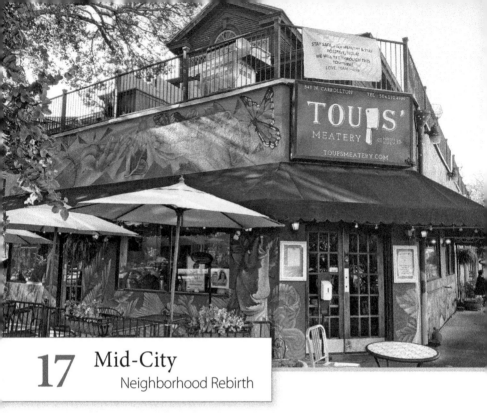

*Above: Award-winning chef Isaac Toups opened his meat-lover's café in 2012.*

BOUNDARIES: Canal St., N. Carrollton Ave., Orleans Ave., City Park Ave.
DISTANCE: 2.4 miles
PARKING: Free on the street
PUBLIC TRANSIT: Canal Streetcar
   (Cemeteries and City Park/Museum Lines)

Like so many neighborhoods in New Orleans, Mid-City was barely recognizable after Hurricane Katrina in 2005. Levee breaches caused extensive flooding to homes and businesses, leaving residents wondering whether their beloved community could survive the devastation.

Not only did it survive, it made one of the most successful comebacks of any New Orleans neighborhood, thanks to the spirit and will of its residents—and a whole slew of volunteers—whose determination to rebuild made it one of the most enviable parts of town.

As its name suggests, Mid-City is the true heart of New Orleans. Listed on the National Register of Historic Places, it consists mostly of structures built in the late 19th and early 20th centuries. The residential section largely consists of bungalows, Creole cottages, and shotguns—narrow homes with rooms arranged one behind the other. And while Mid-City has long had a bustling commercial zone, Katrina rebuilding has given the area a whole new energy and vibe, especially on North Carrollton Avenue between Canal Street and Dumaine Street.

Of course, a New Orleans neighborhood wouldn't be complete without a festival, and one of the best is the Mid-City Bayou Boogaloo, another post-Katrina achievement. In fact, the festival began just a few months after Katrina to help revitalize the area and bring respite and joy to those struggling to rebuild. It has been growing in size and quality ever since.

# Walk Description

Begin at Canal and North Saint Patrick Streets in front of Success Prep @ Thurgood Marshall, a K–8 charter school. Across Canal from Success Prep is St. Anthony of Padua Catholic Church, one of dozens of churches of the Archdiocese of New Orleans.

Facing Canal Street, turn left and walk three blocks to North Alexander Street. The big yellow house on the corner is the ① Ronald McDonald House, which provides a "home away from home" for families with children suffering from cancer. Opened in 1983, it is one of nearly 340 such houses around the world. Among other things, the house offers comfortable beds, laundry and shower facilities, playrooms, and warm meals, most prepared by a dedicated corps of volunteers.

Walk one block to North Hennessey Street. The bright-blue building you'll pass on your left is ② Blue Dot Donuts (4301 Canal), notable for being founded by three New Orleans police officers. Boasting more than 50 kinds of doughnuts, it's been featured on the Cooking Channel and the Food Network.

Continue walking down Canal to North Carrollton Avenue. During this stretch, you'll pass ③ Church Alley Coffee Bar, whose mission is to "empower a more peaceful, resilient, and connected Gulf Coast through forward-thinking products and services," and ④ Café Minh, an upscale Vietnamese restaurant offering such dishes as miso scallops, slow-braised Asian short ribs, and lacquered duck.

Turn left at North Carrollton. If you're hungry or just in the mood for a drink, the next two blocks offer an array of choices. Among other ethnic cuisines, you'll find Italian, Chinese, Mexican, and Japanese. There's ⑤ Zasu, the quaint bistro run by award-winning chef Sue Zemanick; ⑥ Venezia, an old-school Italian restaurant that's been in business since 1957; and ⑦ Revel Cafe & Bar, whose bartender Chris McMillan was named by *Imbibe* magazine as "one of the top 25 most influential cocktail personalities of the last century."

⑧ **Wit's Inn** is a sports bar with some surprisingly tasty pizza. ⑨ **Brown Butter Southern Kitchen & Bar** is the place to go if you're craving such fare as fried pickles, smoked brisket, and crab mac and cheese.

Wherever you go, save room for dessert. ⑩ **Angelo Brocato's**, with its homemade gelato, cannolis, and other Italian pastries, is a must. The old-fashioned ice-cream parlor is a replica of the one the Brocato family opened in Sicily in the early 20th century. At the corner of North Carrollton and Bienville is ⑪ **Bevi Seafood Company**, a seafood shop with some of the tastiest boiled crawfish in town. (Crawfish season runs from early March through the end of June.)

Continue walking down North Carrollton. Between Bienville and St. Louis Streets is Mid-City Market, a commercial development that consists largely of chains such as Panera Bread, Five Guys, and Pinkberry, but you'll also find local favorites, such as ⑫ **Mr. Ed's Oyster Bar and Fish House** and ⑬ **Felipe's Mexican Taqueria**.

Adjacent to Mid-City Market, at St. Louis Street, is a segment of the ⑭ **Lafitte Greenway**, a 2.6-mile multiuse trail and linear park connecting the French Quarter to Bayou St. John and Mid-City. (For more on the greenway, see Walk 18.) From the greenway, walk three blocks to Dumaine Street. Just ahead is ⑮ **Blue Oak BBQ**, which after years of running the kitchen in a local music club has become one of the city's go-to spots for ribs, wings, and brisket. Adjacent to Blue Oak is ⑯ **Parkview Tavern**, which has a dog-friendly patio and lots of TVs for cheering on the Saints.

Cross North Carrollton at Dumaine, where to your right you may notice a line of folks eagerly waiting to place their orders at ⑰ **Pandora's**, one of the oldest snowball stands in New Orleans. On the other side of Dumaine is ⑱ **Toups' Meatery**, where popular chef and *Top Chef* alum Isaac Toups serves up dishes that reflect his Cajun heritage, everything from lamb neck and confit chicken thighs to hot fried quail and boudin balls.

Walk one block back to Orleans Avenue and turn right. Except for a school and a day-care center, this is a residential area known mostly for its Endymion parade celebrations. The Krewe of Endymion, with its dazzling double-decker floats, is one of the most spectacular parades of the Mardi Gras season, and throngs of revelers crowd the Orleans Avenue neutral ground in anticipation. The parade begins at Orleans and City Park Avenue and travels all the way to the Superdome for the Endymion Extravaganza, a star-studded afterparty. But it's along this stretch of Orleans where the real partying takes place: The area is in such demand for parade viewing that many folks camp out days ahead of time to ensure they have a prime spot.

From North Carrollton walk eight blocks to City Park Avenue. To the right is ⓲ City Park (see Walk 19), which at 1,300 acres is one of the largest urban parks in the United States. Across City Park Avenue is ⓳ Delgado Community College, Louisiana's oldest and largest two-year college. Delgado offers 35 associate-degree programs, dozens of certificate and technical-diploma programs, and more than 100 noncredit courses. The largest programs include nursing, general studies, criminal justice, computer information technology, and culinary arts.

Turn left at City Park Avenue. Across from Delgado is a commercial strip that includes ⓴ Ike's Snowballs and ㉒ MoPho, a Southeast Asian café whose chef, Michael Gulotta, once worked in the kitchen of Restaurant August, one of the Crescent City's top-rated restaurants. Pepper jelly–braised clams, crispy chicken wings, and pork-shoulder spring rolls are among its heavenly menu offerings.

Just past the strip, feel free to veer left onto North Anthony Street, where one block down you'll find ㉓ Tubby & Coo's Mid-City Book Shop, the self-described "Nerd Mecca of New Orleans." The shop specializes in such genres as sci-fi and fantasy (think Harry Potter, Dungeons and Dragons, and Doctor Who). Tubby & Coo's prides itself on being "a space where nerds of all shapes and sizes can discover new books and board games and hang out in a space that is welcoming and accepting."

Return to City Park Avenue but be extra-cautious, as parts of the sidewalk are broken up. In a block, you'll be entering one of the largest collections of ㉔ cemeteries in New Orleans. Often referred to as "cities of the dead" because of their aboveground grave sites, they include the Masonic, Cypress Grove, Greenwood, and St. Patrick's. Turn left at Canal Street and you'll encounter Odd Fellow's Rest, the Charity Hospital Cemetery, and a Jewish cemetery. Each cemetery has its own fascinating background. Cypress Grove, for example, was the first cemetery built to honor the city's volunteer firefighters and their families. Odd Fellow's was built to provide a burial site for Protestant African Americans, who were barred from being buried with whites. The Charity Hospital Cemetery features a ㉕ Hurricane Katrina Memorial, along with mausoleums that hold the remains of those whose bodies were unclaimed after the storm.

At the corner of City Park Avenue and Canal Boulevard are two of the Crescent City's favorites: ㉖ Morning Call, where hot fried beignets and café au lait top the menu, and ㉗ Bud's Broiler, part of a locally owned burger chain that's been around since the 1950s. Try the burger with grated cheddar and smoked hickory sauce, and be sure to add an order of onion rings and a chocolate milkshake. (Make sure to save room for beignets!)

As you head back to your starting point on North St. Patrick, you'll pass ㉘ Sacred Grinds, which as a self-described "haunted" coffee house is the perfect fit for this neighborhood of cemeteries.

Just down the block is the ㉙ Beachcorner Bar & Grill, a burger joint and sports bar. Take note of the Victorian mansion across Canal at the corner of St. Bernadotte Street. Built as a private residence in 1872 by Mary Slattery and renovated in subsequent years by various other owners, the mansion served as P. J. McMahon & Sons Funeral Home from 1930 to 1985. It is now used as a special-events venue and, come October, as the ㉚ Mortuary Haunted House—known for being so spooky that those under 18 are discouraged from visiting. During the year, paranormal experts lead ghost tours and ghost hunting investigations, sharing "the secret legendary history of the mansion and why some of the souls that passed through the home never left."

## Points of Interest

1. Ronald McDonald House  rmhc-nola.org, 4403 Canal St., 504-486-6668

2. Blue Dot Donuts  facebook.com/bluedotdonuts, 4301 Canal St., 504-218-4866

3. Church Alley Coffee Bar  churchalleycoffeebar.com, 4201 Canal St., 504-304-6306

4. Café Minh  cafeminh.com, 4139 Canal St., 504-482-6266

5. Zasu  zasunola.com, 127 N. Carrollton Ave., 504-267-3233

6. Venezia  venezianeworleans.net, 134 N. Carrollton Ave., 504-488-7991

7. Revel Cafe & Bar  revelcafeandbar.com, 133 N. Carrollton Ave., 504-309-6122

8. Wit's Inn  witsinn.com, 141 N. Carrollton Ave., 504-486-1600

9. Brown Butter Southern Kitchen & Bar  brownbutterrestaurant.com, 231 N. Carrollton Ave., 504-609-3871

10. Angelo Brocato's  angelobrocatoicecream.com, 214 N. Carrollton Ave., 504-486-1465

11. Bevi Seafood Company  beviseafoodco.com, 236 N. Carrollton Ave., 504-488-7503

12. Mr. Ed's Oyster Bar and Fish House  mredsrestaurants.com, 301 N. Carrollton Ave., 504-872-9975

13. Felipe's Mexican Taqueria  felipestaqueria.com, 411-1 N. Carrollton Ave., 504-408-2626

14. Lafitte Greenway  lafittegreenway.org, Basin Street to Canal Boulevard, 504-462-0645

15. Blue Oak BBQ  blueoakbbq.com, 900 N. Carrollton Ave., 504-822-2583

16. Parkview Tavern  910 N. Carrollton Ave., 504-482-2680

17. Pandora's  facebook.com/PandorasSnowballs, 901 N. Carrollton Ave., 504-285-4867

18. Toups' Meatery  toupsmeatery.com, 845 N. Carrollton Ave., 504-252-4999

19. City Park  neworleanscitypark.com, 1 Palm Drive, 504-482-4888

20. Delgado Community College  dcc.edu, 615 City Park Ave., 504-671-5000

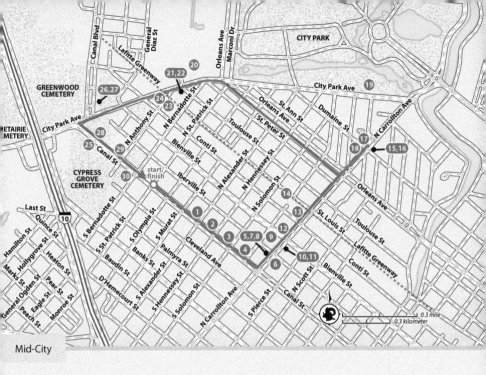

Mid-City

- 21 Ike's Snowballs  ikessnowballs.com, 520 City Park Ave., 504-208-9983
- 22 MoPho  mophonola.com, 514 City Park Ave., 504-482-6845
- 23 Tubby & Coo's Mid-City Book Shop  tubbyandcoos.com, 432 St. Anthony St., 504-345-8491
- 24 Cemeteries  saveourcemeteries.org, 504-525-3377
- 25 Hurricane Katrina Memorial  5056 Canal St.
- 26 Morning Call  morningcallcoffeestand.com, 5101 Canal Blvd.
- 27 Bud's Broiler  budsbroiler.com, 5101 Canal Blvd.
- 28 Sacred Grinds  facebook.com/zombiejesu, 5055 Canal St., 504-488-4889
- 29 Beachcorner Bar & Grill  beachcornerbarandgrill.com, 4905 Canal St., 504-488-7357
- 30 Mortuary Haunted House  themortuary.net, 4800 Canal St., 504-483-2350

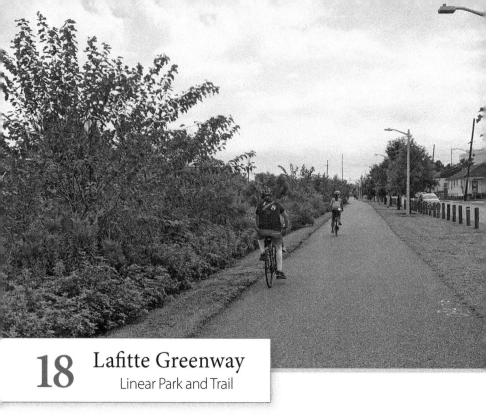

# 18 Lafitte Greenway
## Linear Park and Trail

BOUNDARIES: North Alexander St., St. Louis St., Basin St.
DISTANCE: 2.6 miles
PARKING: Street parking
PUBLIC TRANSIT: Canal Street streetcar

When the Lafitte Greenway opened in 2015, it was the culmination of years of grassroots support to transform what was once a railroad corridor into a public green space for bikers and pedestrians.

The opening of the 2.6-mile linear park that connects Mid-City with the French Quarter was met with great fanfare, and it has become a popular alternative to the Crescent City's other parks ever since.

Although managed by the New Orleans Recreation Department, the Friends of the Lafitte Greenway deserves most of the credit for initiating the idea of such a space. The nonprofit formed in 2006, the year after Hurricane Katrina destroyed much of the city. Community activists saw an opportunity to reimagine New Orleans, and a public green space that offered economic, environmental, health, and cultural benefits was high atop their wish list.

The park stretches from the Alexander Street Trailhead to the Basin Street Station and includes various stopping points along the way. During your walk, you can grab a beer at the Wrong Iron, a po'boy at Parkway Bakery & Tavern, or a glass of wine at the Bayou Wine Garden. Art installations such as sculptures and murals abound along the Greenway, and if you time your walk right, you can even partake in a yoga or kickboxing class on the Greenway Great Lawn.

Every year, the Greenway holds a variety of family-friendly events, including an arts and music festival, a Halloween Spooktacular, and an Easter Eggstravaganza.

Bear in mind that the walk described here is one way. You can double your mileage and steps by making an about-face at the end and returning to the starting point by foot. Otherwise, you can take a taxi or ride-sharing service back. If you're with a group, you may even want to arrange to park a car at the end.

## Walk Description

Begin your walk on the ❶ Lafitte Greenway at the North Alexander Trailhead at the intersection of North Alexander and St. Louis Streets. Walk four blocks to North Carrollton Avenue, a bustling area that features such eateries as ❷ Felipe's Mexican Taqueria and ❸ Mr. Ed's Oyster Bar & Fish House. Just before you hit North Carrollton, look for the colorful *Tree of Life* mural near the ❹ Massey's Outfitters loading dock. The mural is the work of artist Rick Sinnett, whose inspiration for the piece is the Susie Tree that survived the 1995 Oklahoma City bombing.

Cross Carrollton and continue walking toward the next main intersection at North Norman C. Francis Parkway. Consider a stop at the ❺ Wrong Iron, located just off the Greenway on Toulouse Street. This lively beer garden has become one of the city's go-to venues for watching Saints and LSU games. The Wrong Iron boasts 50 beers, 10 wines, five cocktails, and four frozen drinks on tap, and there are always one or two food trucks providing sustenance.

Just ahead, at the intersection of the Greenway and Norman C. Francis Parkway, is an installation titled *Turning (Prayer Wheels for the Mississippi River)* by artist Michael Varisco. The sculpture features three 9-foot stainless steel cylinders, or "prayer wheels," representing three periods of the river's history—the wild era, colonial planation era, and petrochemical era. The bases of each cylinder feature mosaics that depict the land-building patterns created from deposits of the river's sediment. Visitors are invited to spin the cylinders to emit blue light.

Other stopping points at this location include ⑥ **Parkway Bakery and Tavern,** just to your left on Hagan Avenue, ⑦ **Bayou Beer Garden** to your right on Norman C. Francis, and ⑧ **Bayou Wine Garden** on North Rendon Street. In a city that boasts one great po'boy joint after the other, Parkway consistently ranks at the top, its sloppy roast beef creations billed as "comfort food at its finest." But don't let the name "bakery" fool you. Although Parkway opened in 1911 as a neighborhood bake shop, today's Parkway is all about the po'boy, and not just roast beef. Po'boys include shrimp, oyster, catfish, meatball, and alligator sausage.

Continue down the Greenway to the next major intersection at North Broad Street. Just to your left on North Broad is ⑨ **The Broad Theater,** a cool independent movie house that shows mainstream as well as indie flicks and documentaries. The Broad has its own bar, where you can choose among a variety of drinks whether you plan to see a movie or not.

On the next five blocks, between North Broad and North Galvez Streets, you'll pass the Greenway's tennis courts, a playground, and the FitLot Fitness Park, one of two exercise venues that offer free and accessible fitness equipment to the community. Look for the *Paul Pogba* mural by artist Brandon "BMike" Odums about three blocks down, to your right, on North Rocheblave at St. Louis Street. The mural features soccer star Paul Pogba of Manchester United and the French National Team and is one of three *Larger Than Life* murals nationwide featuring three soccer superstars in honor of the World Cup.

Just past North Galvez, the trail winds through the Greenway Great Lawn, where you might see a yoga class, hip-hop kickboxing class, or body weight boot camp in action. Your stroll will also take you past a football and soccer field, a baseball field, a basketball court, another playground, and the Lemann Pool. Outside the pool building you'll see another wall mural, this one by artist Keith Duncan and the Young Artists Movement (YAM). The *Peace & Unity* mural came about through a series of community conversations about racial reconciliation. To your right, on an aluminum building near North Roman Street, is another BMike mural, this one celebrating the history of the city's Coliseum Arena, which once stood at this location. Closed since 1960, the arena hosted boxing matches and other sporting events, musical performances, and speeches, including one by Dr. Martin Luther King in 1957.

Just past the playground, cross North Claiborne. To your left, under the I-10 overpass, is ⑩ **Veggienola,** a juice bar and health food café that specializes in the Bissap Breeze, a beverage that combines organic roselle hibiscus flowers, volcanic agave nectar, and fresh ginger and cinnamon.

After crossing North Claiborne, continue on the last segment of the Greenway, which features another playground and basketball court. The trail continues along Basin Street and ends at the Basin Street Trailhead, just in front of ⑪ **Basin St. Station,** a visitor center featuring community exhibits, a performance venue, a walking tour kiosk, and a gift shop.

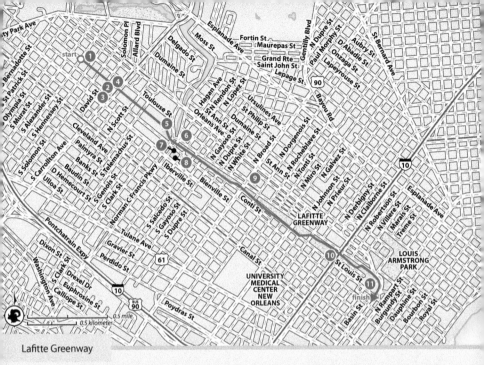

Lafitte Greenway

## Points of Interest

1. Lafitte Greenway  lafittegreenway.org, 2200 Lafitte Ave., 504-462-0645

2. Felipe's Mexican Taqueria  felipestaqueria.com, 411-1 N. Carrollton Ave., 504-408-2626

3. Mr. Ed's Oyster Bar & Fish House  mredsrestaurants.com 301 N. Carrollton Ave., 504-872-9975

4. Massey's Outfitters  masseysoutfitters.com, 509 N. Carrollton Ave., 504-648-0292

5. Wrong Iron  wrongiron.com, 3523 Toulouse St., 504-302-0528

6. Parkway Bakery and Tavern  parkwaypoorboys.com, 538 Hagan Ave., 504-482-3047

7. Bayou Beer Garden  bayoubeergarden.com, 326 N. Norman C. Francis Pkwy., 504-302-9357

8. Bayou Wine Garden  bayouwinegarden.com, 315 N. Rendon St., 504-826-2925

9. The Broad Theater  thebroadtheater.com, 636 N. Broad St., 504-218-1008

10. Veggienola  veggienola.com, underneath I-10 bridge at N. Claiborne Ave., 504-515-1233

11. Basin St. Station  basinststation.com, 501 Basin St., 504-293-2600

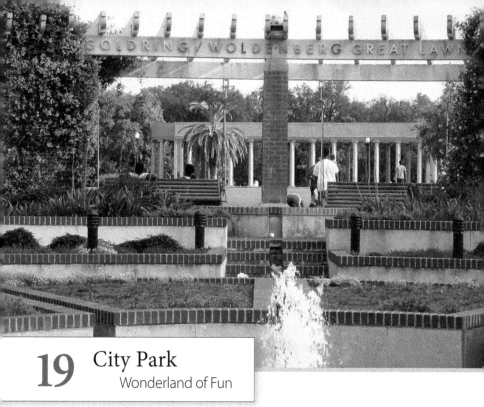

# 19 City Park
## Wonderland of Fun

BOUNDARIES: City Park Ave., Marconi Dr., Wisner Blvd., Victory Ave.
DISTANCE: 1.47 miles
PARKING: Free on the street or in the park
PUBLIC TRANSIT: Canal Streetcar (City Park/Museum Line)

City Park is a 1,300-acre wonderland—and Hurricane Katrina spared none of it. The storm and subsequent federal levee breaches flooded one of the country's largest and oldest urban parks, leaving sections of it with up to 8 feet of water and causing $43 million in damage.

Fast-forward 15 years, and the park is better than ever, thanks to the dedication of volunteers from around the country and Friends of City Park, the park's fundraising arm. Back are most of the park's treasured staples, from the New Orleans Botanical Garden and Storyland to Carousel

Gardens and the New Orleans Museum of Art, including the Sydney and Walda Besthoff Sculpture Garden. Its trees are as magnificent as ever, despite the park having lost 2,000 of them in the storm.

Attractions include City Putt, a 36-hole miniature golf course; the Goldring-Woldenberg Great Lawn, a vast green space used for concerts and other activities; and the stunning Big Lake, with its surrounding bike and jogging paths. It is also the new home of the Louisiana Children's Museum, which unlike its previous Warehouse District location features an expansive outdoor area with an edible garden, a floating classroom, and a tree trunk trail.

If that weren't enough, the park is also home to two of the Crescent City's premier events: the Voodoo Music Experience in October and Celebration in the Oaks, one of the country's most spectacular holiday-lights festivals. Since 2008, City Park has also been the site of such movies and TV shows as *The Expendables, Now You See Me,* and *22 Jump Street.*

Bear in mind that this walk covers only a section of the park. Feel free to explore its other gems, such as the Popp Fountain, the disc-golf course, the NOLA City Bark dog park, and the Couturie Forest and Arboretum, on your own. The park also features a tennis center, a golf course, an equestrian farm, and a fishing pier. *Note:* Some roads in the park aren't marked, so bring along this book and/or the official park map, available at neworleanscitypark.com/in-the-park/city-park-map.

# Walk Description

Begin your walk at North Hennessey Street and City Park Avenue. Take note of the trees, especially the majestic, moss-dripping live oaks, which ❶ City Park considers its pride and joy. The park boasts the oldest grove of mature live oaks in the world, and some—like the McDonogh and Anseman Oaks—are approximately 600–800 years old. Although City Park lost 2,000 of its 20,000 trees in Katrina, more than 5,000 new trees have been planted since. In addition to live oaks, you'll see bald cypress, magnolia, and other tree species. Feel free to wander through the maze of trees and take a closer look. You'll be glad you did.

Return to the walkway and, facing City Park Avenue, turn right, then walk one block to Anseman Avenue. Enter the park on Anseman through the Pizzati Gate, and cross the Anseman Bridge over Bayou Metairie, one of the many lagoons that wind through the park. The bridge, built in 1938 to replace the original 1928 structure, is named in honor of Victor Anseman, who, as the park's first executive committee chairman and volunteer manager, earned the title "Father of City Park."

At Dreyfous Drive, turn right and continue walking past two of the park's most historic landmarks: the Peristyle and the Popp Bandstand. The Peristyle, a Neoclassical open-air pavilion with a colonnade, was built in 1907 as a party place. It has undergone numerous renovations over the years, and today it is one of the park's most popular wedding and photo-taking venues. The Classical Greek–style Popp Bandstand went up in 1917. Designed by noted New Orleans architect Emile Weil, it features 12 granite columns topped with a bronze dome. In its infancy, it served as an outdoor theater for some of the earliest moving pictures, and dozens of musicians, including John Philip Sousa, have performed here over the years. Between the Peristyle and Popp Bandstand is the Stanley Ray Playground, which features swings, slides, and climbing contraptions.

Across from the Peristyle is the Goldring-Woldenberg Great Lawn, a 3-acre green space that opened in 2010 as part of the park's master plan. Adorned with palms, brick pathways, swings, pavilions, and a fountain, the lawn is frequently the site of concerts such as the Louisiana Philharmonic Orchestra's annual Swing in the Oaks.

Continue down Dreyfous past the Casino Building, a Spanish Mission–style structure built in 1913. Today, it's home to the famous ❷ **Café Du Monde**, known for its café au lait and sugar-laden beignets.

Continue on Dreyfous, cross the bridge, and turn left onto Dueling Oaks Drive. This will take you to Collins Diboll Circle, adjacent to the ❸ **New Orleans Museum of Art**. At the circle, turn right; then make another right onto Lelong Drive, walk to the end of the block, and cross Lelong in front of the park's Wisner Boulevard entrance. Walk back toward the museum on the other side of Lelong. To your right is Big Lake, which opened in 2009, providing park-goers with yet another opportunity for recreation. The lake is surrounded by 25 acres of wildlife and wetlands and paths for jogging, walking, and biking. Both boats and bikes are available to rent.

Consider a stop at the New Orleans Museum of Art, which boasts a permanent collection of nearly 40,000 objects. The museum is especially known for its French and American art, along with photography, glass, and African and Japanese works. It is also a popular venue for films, plays, lectures, children's art workshops, wellness activities, and live-music performances.

Circle right around the museum, past Big Lake and onto Roosevelt Mall. (Be sure to follow a map because some streets aren't marked.) Cross the bridge and continue walking down the right side of Roosevelt Mall. One of the highlights of this stretch is the ❹ **Louisiana Children's Museum**, an 8.5-acre play space where kids can explore, discover, and learn to their hearts' content. The museum features both indoor and outdoor exhibits that, among other things, invite children to view the park's wildlife through binoculars, build a levee or dam at the Sedimentation Station, learn about Louisiana food in a kid-size kitchen, and go on a New Orleans–themed scavenger hunt. When you need a break, Acorn is a Dickie Brennan café that offers dishes for big and little appetites.

Continue down Roosevelt Mall and make a U-turn at the next intersection. Turn left and walk on the other side of Roosevelt Mall to Victory Avenue. Turn right on Victory, where to your left

## Sydney and Walda Besthoff Sculpture Garden

No matter where your eyes take you in the Sydney and Walda Besthoff Sculpture Garden at City Park, beauty abounds. An extension of the New Orleans Museum of Art, the 11-acre garden comprises more than 90 sculptures situated among winding footpaths, reflecting lagoons, ancient live oaks, and pedestrian bridges. Among them are Robert Indiana's *Love, Red Blue;* Henry Moore's *Reclining Mother and Child;* Pierre-Auguste Renoir's *Venus Victorious;* and George Rodrigue's *Blue Dog.* Other contemporary artists whose works are represented in the garden include Ida Kohlmeyer, Gaston Lachaise, Jean-Michel Othoniel, Yaacov Agam, and Joel Shapiro.

Open since 2003 and doubled in size in 2019, the sculpture garden is named for New Orleans philanthropists and art collectors Sydney and Walda Besthoff, who through their private foundation donated most of the works that fill the garden. The foundation is dedicated to cultivating public interest in contemporary sculpture, and the garden—free and open to the public seven days a week—has served as a conduit to fulfilling that mission.

The museum offers a free audio tour accessible though visitors' cell phones. Additional programming includes yoga and Tai Chi classes, school field trips, and a spring Easter-egg hunt.

---

is the 11-acre ⑤ **Sydney and Walda Besthoff Sculpture Garden,** considered one of the most important sculpture installations in the United States (see sidebar above).

From the sculpture garden, continue down Victory past the ⑥ **New Orleans Botanical Garden.** What began as the City Park Rose Garden in 1936 is today home to 2,000 varieties of plants from around the world, among them aquatics, roses, native plants, ornamental trees, shrubs, and perennials. Highlights include the New Orleans Historic Train Garden, the Yakumo Nihon Teien Japanese Garden, the Conservatory of the Two Sisters, the Pavilion of the Two Sisters, the Garden Study Center, the Lath House, and the Robert B. Haspel Stage. The Botanical Garden presents a variety of programming throughout the year, including garden shows, lectures, and concerts, such as "Thursdays at Twilight," a garden concert series that showcases some of the city's top musicians and bands. The outdoor Kitchen in the Garden offers a variety of healthy cooking programs and on Wednesday evenings hosts boxed meal picnics.

Next to the Botanical Garden is the park's iconic ⑦ **Storyland,** a must-see playground filled with fairy-tale sculptures such as Humpty Dumpty, the Three Little Pigs, and the Cheshire Cat. Kids are invited to climb aboard Captain Hook's pirate ship, follow Pinocchio into the mouth of a whale, and race up Jack and Jill's Hill.

Adjacent to Storyland is ⑧ **Carousel Gardens,** an amusement park with 16 rides, including an antique wooden carousel that dates back to 1906. The carousel has 56 animals (mostly flying

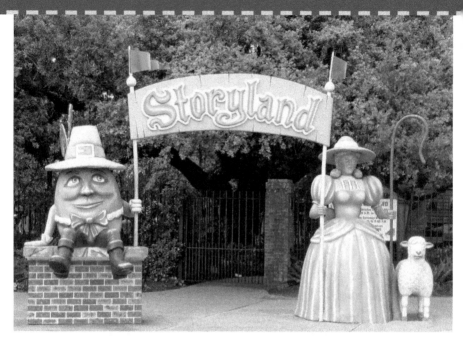

*Humpty Dumpty and Little Bo Peep greet guests at City Park's Storyland.*

horses) and two chariots. Listed on the National Register of Historic Places, it is one of only 100 hand-carved carousels in the United States and the only one in Louisiana. Other rides include bumper cars, a Tilt-A-Whirl, a Ferris wheel, the Musik Express, and a miniature train. Kiddie rides are available for the toddler set.

Across from Carousel Gardens is **9 City Putt**, a 36-hole miniature-golf complex with two courses. The Louisiana Course focuses on themes and cities from around the state; the New Orleans Course showcases streets and local icons such as Louis Armstrong and Mr. Bingle, a storied Christmas character (a snowman with an ice-cream-cone hat) associated with the old Maison Blanche department store.

Continue down Victory two blocks to Stadium Drive and turn left. Walk another block back to Dreyfous and turn left. Take Dreyfous to Anseman, turn right, and exit the park. Turn left and return to the starting point.

Though not part of the park, **10 Ralph's on the Park**, directly across the street from the Anseman entrance, is yet another of the city's classy eateries. It's an upscale restaurant, so if you're not quite dressed for it, do consider it another time.

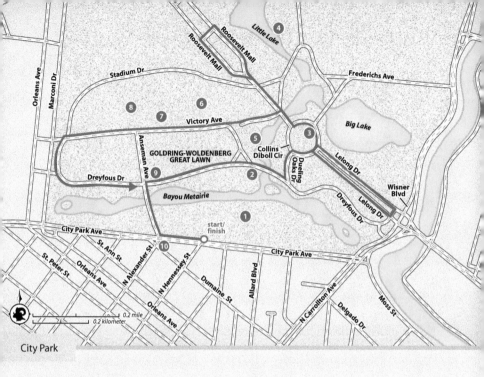

City Park

## Points of Interest

1. City Park  neworleanscitypark.com, 1 Palm Drive, 504-482-4888

2. Café Du Monde  cafedumonde.com, 56 Dreyfous Drive, 504-766-0250

3. New Orleans Museum of Art  noma.org, 1 Collins Diboll Circle, 504-658-4100

4. Louisiana Children's Museum  lcm.org, 15 Henry Thomas Drive, 504-523-1357

5. Sydney and Walda Besthoff Sculpture Garden  noma.org, 1 Collins Diboll Circle, 504-658-4100

6. New Orleans Botanical Garden  neworleanscitypark.com/botanical-garden, 3 Victory Ave., 504-483-4888

7. Storyland  neworleanscitypark.com/in-the-park/storyland, 7 Victory Ave., 504-483-4888

8. Carousel Gardens Amusement Park  neworleanscitypark.com/in-the-park/carousel-gardens, 7 Victory Avenue, 504-483-9402

9. City Putt  neworleanscitypark.com/in-the-park/city-putt, 8 Victory Ave., 504-483-9385

10. Ralph's on the Park  ralphsonthepark.com, 900 City Park Ave., 504-488-1000

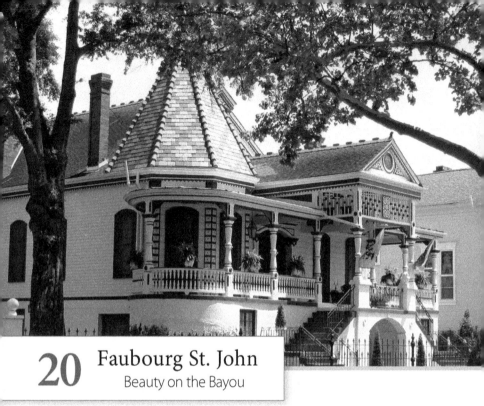

## 20 Faubourg St. John
### Beauty on the Bayou

*Above: The Cresson House is just one of many stunning homes that line Esplanade Avenue.*

BOUNDARIES: Esplanade Ave., N. White St., Grand Route St. John, Moss St.
DISTANCE: 1.66 miles
PARKING: Free street parking
PUBLIC TRANSIT: Canal Streetcar (City Park/Museum Line)

Faubourg St. John, a section of the Esplanade Ridge Historic District, is one of those neighborhoods that, once you call it home, will likely be home forever. This community has it all, from stunning Creole cottages and Victorian mansions to parks, restaurants, cafés, and museums.

It is also a tight-knit community that, through the Faubourg St. John Neighborhood Association, has participated in numerous beautification projects, among them playground and park improvements, tree plantings, and neutral-ground maintenance.

Faubourg St. John dates back to 1708—10 years before the city of New Orleans was founded—when the French entered the city via Bayou St. John, which is connected to Lake

Pontchartrain by way of the Gulf of Mexico and the Mississippi River. It eventually became the neighborhood of choice for the area's upper-class Creoles, particularly on Esplanade Avenue, an oak- and sycamore-lined street that stretches 2.5 miles from the river to City Park.

Just steps away from Bayou St. John and City Park, Faubourg St. John is within walking distance of such festivals as Bayou Boogaloo, held annually along Bayou St. John, and the New Orleans Jazz & Heritage Festival, held every year on the last weekend in April and the first weekend in May at the nearby Fair Grounds Race Course.

## Walk Description

Begin at ❶ St. Louis Cemetery No. 3, established in 1854, when a yellow fever outbreak drove the need for more burial space. The cemetery is home to a number of "society tombs" owned by fraternal organizations, including those of the Dante Lodge of Masons, the Young Men's Benevolent Association, and the United Slavonian Benevolent Association. Before it was a cemetery, the site was a leper colony known as "Leper's Land."

Across the street is ❷ Desmare Playground, one of the city's many neighborhood parks and playgrounds. Desmare has undergone numerous facelifts over the years, many of them courtesy of members of the Faubourg St. John Neighborhood Association, which holds annual fundraisers to help its cause. Future plans include additional playground equipment and an educational Rain Garden to show how New Orleans can better live with water.

Walk one block to ❸ Cabrini High School, a Catholic girls' school named for St. Frances Xavier Cabrini, the first woman to establish a missionary order of women and the first American citizen to be canonized as a saint of the Catholic Church. The school opened in 1959 in what was then the Sacred Heart Orphan Asylum. Mother Cabrini raised the money for both the orphanage and the school, once saying, "The greatest heritage to a girl is a good education."

Next to Cabrini is the back of ❹ Our Lady of the Rosary Catholic Church, founded in 1907. The church, which faces Bayou St. John, had its majestic copper dome replated after Hurricane Katrina, and the dome is illuminated at night.

If you'd like, take a brief detour left on Leda Court, where about a half block down you'll find the massive ❺ Luling Mansion, a historical landmark that was once one of the most grandiose homes in New Orleans. Now divided into apartments, the Italian Renaissance mansion was designed in 1865 by renowned architect James Gallier for cotton merchant Florence Luling. It later served as the home of the Louisiana Jockey Club before it was sold to private owners in 1905.

From Leda Court, continue walking down Esplanade. The next stretch of blocks features two family-owned grocery stores, ❻ Terranova's Supermarket and ❼ Canseco's, the latter of which makes the same delectable Cuban sandwiches sold at the New Orleans Jazz and Heritage Festival. The area is also abundant with restaurants—⑧ Lola's, known for its paella and other Spanish fare; ⑨ Santa Fe, a Southwestern restaurant offering live jazz on Thursday and Sunday nights; ⑩ Café Degas, a French eatery with one of the best patio dining rooms in town; and ⑪ Nonna Mia, a pizzeria that also serves classic Sicilian pasta dishes. On Ponce de Leon Street, just off Esplanade by Canseco's, you'll find ⑫ 1000 Figs, a Mediterranean eatery; ⑬ Fair Grinds, a coffeehouse that specializes in fair trade coffee, tea, and chocolate; ⑭ Swirl, a wine bar and market; and, at the corner of North Lopez Street, ⑮ Liuzza's by the Track, where the signature dish is the barbecue shrimp po'boy.

From Café Degas, walk four blocks to 2821 Esplanade, a Neo-Tudor–style residence built in the 1920s. Next door, at 2809 Esplanade, is a Queen Anne–style home built in 1902. Known as the Cresson House, it is a favorite photo-taking spot.

Cross Esplanade at North White Street in front of ⑯ ReNEW McDonogh City Park Academy, part of the city's almost all-charter school system. On the opposite side of Esplanade, you'll pass ⑰ CC's Coffee House, a great place to grab a latte or cappuccino. Continue on North White one block to the corner of Bell Street. The DuFour-Plassan House, at 1206 N. White, was built in 1870 and boasts one of the few wrought-iron cornstalk fences in New Orleans.

Turn right on Bell and walk one block to North Dupre Street. Turn right on North Dupre, walk two blocks to Esplanade, and turn left. Walk three blocks to Grand Route St. John. As you walk down Esplanade, you'll notice an array of architectural styles from classic bungalows to Greek Revivals, many adorned with black-and-gold Jazz Fest flags. Because the neighborhood is built on naturally high ground, it escaped the flooding that ravaged so many other New Orleans neighborhoods in Hurricane Katrina.

Turn left onto Grand Route St. John in front of ⑱ Fortier Park, an intimate green space that boasts sculptures, palms, and other lush greenery. The park is named for Alcee Fortier, a philanthropist and professor of romance languages at Tulane University.

Walk four blocks to Moss Street on Grand Route St. John, one of the neighborhood's most beautifully maintained streets. Turn right onto Moss in front of the meandering Bayou St. John. This is believed to be the approximate spot where, back in the 18th and early 19th centuries, travelers disembarked from boats as they made their way into the city via Grand Route St. John. At the corner of Moss and Grand Route St. John is the Old Spanish Custom House, which was built in 1784 and is the oldest building in the neighborhood.

Continue walking down Moss past ⑲ Bayou St. John Bed and Breakfast, a 150-year-old house-turned-inn at 1318 Moss. Another historic structure is the Holy Rosary rectory (1342 Moss), a Greek Revival mansion built in 1834.

As you continue walking, take note of the pedestrian-only bridge that crosses the bayou in front of Cabrini High School. Known as the Magnolia Bridge, it's a popular spot for parties and fishing. Next to Cabrini High, at 1440 Moss, is the ㉑ Pitot House, an 18th-century Creole Colonial plantation that serves as the home of the Louisiana Landmarks Society. The organization works to promote historic preservation through education and advocacy and invites the public to tour the house and learn about life along the bayou since the earliest days of the settlement. Each year, the society hosts a series of fundraisers called Vino on the Bayou, featuring wine tastings, music, and food.

From Pitot House, continue down Moss and circle right as you head back to Esplanade. Across the bayou are ㉑ City Park and the ㉒ New Orleans Museum of Art (see the previous walk). Cross Esplanade, turn right, and return to the starting point at St. Louis Cemetery No. 3.

## Points of Interest

1. St. Louis Cemetery No. 3  saveourcemeteries.org, 3421 Esplanade Ave., 504-482-5065
2. Desmare Playground  3456 Esplanade Ave. between Esplanade and Moss Street
3. Cabrini High School  cabrinihigh.com, 1400 Moss St., 504-482-1193
4. Our Lady of the Rosary Catholic Church  ourladyoftherosary-no.com, 3368 Esplanade Ave., 504-488-2659
5. Luling Mansion  1436 Leda Ct.
6. Terranova's Supermarket  3308 Esplanade Ave., 504-482-4131
7. Canseco's  cansecos.com, 3135 Esplanade Ave., 504-322-2594
8. Lola's  lolasneworleans.com, 3312 Esplanade Ave., 504-488-6946
9. Santa Fe  santafenola.com, 3201 Esplanade Ave., 504-948-0077
10. Café Degas  cafedegas.com, 3127 Esplanade Ave., 504-945-5635
11. Nonna Mia  nonnamia.net, 3125 Esplanade Ave., 504-948-1717
12. 1000 Figs  1000figs.com, 3141 Ponce de Leon St., 504-301-0848
13. Fair Grinds Coffeehouse  fairgrinds.com, 3133 Ponce de Leon St., 504-913-9072
14. Swirl Wine Bar & Market  swirlnola.com, 3143 Ponce de Leon St., 504-304-0635
15. Liuzza's by the Track  liuzzasbythetrack.com, 1518 N. Lopez St., 504-218-7888
16. ReNEW McDonogh City Park Academy  renewschools.org
17. CC's Coffee House  ccscoffee.com, 2800 Esplanade Ave., 504-482-9865

*(continued on next page)*

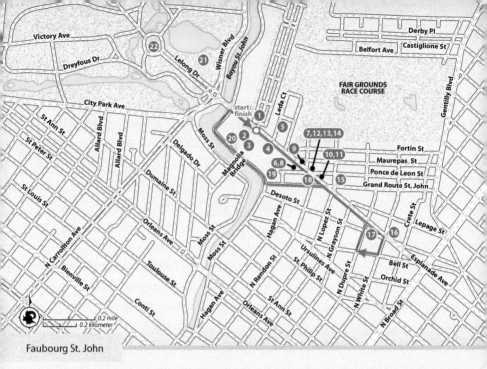

Faubourg St. John

(continued from previous page)

**18** Fortier Park  Bounded by Esplanade Avenue, Grand Route St. John, and Mystery Street

**19** Bayou St. John Bed and Breakfast  1318 Moss St., 504-482-6677

**20** Pitot House  louisianalandmarks.org, 1440 Moss St., 504-482-0312

**21** City Park  neworleanscitypark.com, 1 Palm Drive, 504-482-4888

**22** New Orleans Museum of Art  noma.org, 1 Collins Diboll Circle, 504-658-4100

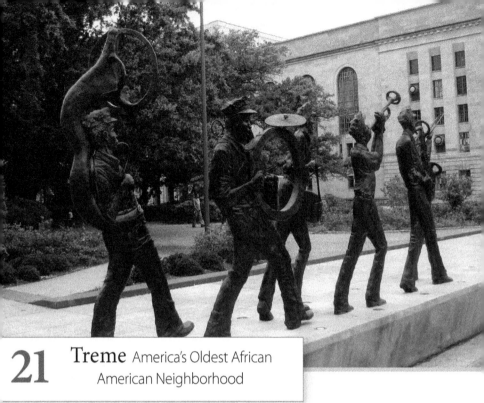

# 21 Treme America's Oldest African American Neighborhood

*Above: These sculptures in Armstrong Park honor the city's rich jazz heritage.*

BOUNDARIES: Basin St., N. Rampart St., Governor Nicholls St., N. Robertson St.
DISTANCE: 1.46 miles
PARKING: Metered parking on N. Rampart St.
PUBLIC TRANSIT: RTA Buses #57 (Franklin), #88 (St. Claude/Jackson Barracks), and #91
  (Jackson-Esplanade)

For countless Mardi Gras revelers, celebrating Fat Tuesday means packing up the family, picking up some Popeye's, and heading to St. Charles Avenue to enjoy a day of parades. For others, it means heading out of town and not returning until the last strand of beads has been tossed.

Then there are those who wouldn't spend the day anywhere else but in Treme (pronounced *treh-MAY*), the oldest African American neighborhood in the United States and the cultural heart of New Orleans. In Treme, Mardi Gras means second-line parades, exquisitely costumed Mardi

Gras Indians, and the North Side Skull and Bones Gang, which has been waking up the neighborhood on Fat Tuesday since 1819.

Unless you're in New Orleans for Mardi Gras, you won't have the chance to experience that exuberating scene. But on any given day in Treme, you might witness a jazz funeral, a spontaneous second-line parade, or a wandering musician blowing his horn just because.

Such scenes played out weekly on the critically acclaimed HBO series *Treme,* which chronicled the struggles of musicians and other residents in the months and years following Katrina. The series lasted only three seasons (2010–2013), but it exposed to the world one of America's most fascinating neighborhoods.

## Walk Description

Begin at Congo Square in ❶ **Louis Armstrong Park.** The 31-acre park includes the New Orleans Municipal Auditorium, the Mahalia Jackson Theater for the Performing Arts, and Congo Square, where in the 18th century slaves would gather on Sundays—their day off—to set up market and play music. In addition to walking paths, lagoons, and gardens, the park contains a statue of Armstrong, a bust of jazz saxophonist Sidney Bechet, and a sculpture of Buddy Bolden, a cornetist often referred to as the Father of Jazz. As one might expect, the park is home to numerous music festivals, including the Louisiana Cajun-Zydeco Festival and Jazz in the Park, a series of concerts featuring such greats as the Treme Brass Band, Irma Thomas, and Charmaine Neville.

Across the street and down the block on North Rampart are two of this area's trendiest bars, ❷ **Bar Tonique** and ❸ **Effervescence.** Bar Tonique boasts a menu of original, adapted, and classic cocktails, along with eclectic beer and wine selections. Effervescence is a sparkling wine lounge that offers three types of caviar, among other bites.

At North Rampart and Dumaine is the site of the old J&M Recording Studio, considered the birthplace of rhythm and blues. Among the greats who recorded there were local luminaries Fats Domino and Aaron Neville, as well as stars such as Little Richard, Jerry Lee Lewis, and Ray Charles.

Walk to the end of the park, then another block to Ursulines Avenue, and turn left. Walk one block to Henriette Delille Street and turn right. This street is named for the founder of the Catholic order of the Sisters of the Holy Family in New Orleans. Delille, a free woman of color, devoted her life to serving the poor.

In the middle of the block is the ❹ **Backstreet Cultural Museum,** which opened in 1999 to preserve and perpetuate the cultural traditions of New Orleans's African American community. The museum has the world's most comprehensive collection of artifacts related to the masking

# St. Augustine Catholic Church

The oldest African American Catholic parish in the United States, St. Augustine was established on the property of a one-time plantation as the result of a decision by Bishop Antoine Blanc to allow free people of color a place to worship.

One of the more fascinating stories about the church is the so-called War of the Pews. Just before the church was dedicated in 1842, people of color began buying pews for their family members. White people responded by buying their own pews, their goal to buy more than the "colored" members. Their campaign failed, for the free people of color ended up buying three pews to every one bought by the whites. In what the church described as an unprecedented social, political, and religious move, the free people of color also bought the pews of both side-aisles and gave them to the slaves as their exclusive place of worship, a first in the history of slavery in the United States. According to the church's website, the mix of the pews resulted in the most integrated congregation in the United States.

In 2004, St. Augustine dedicated the Tomb of the Unknown Slave, described on a bronze plaque as a "shrine consisting of grave crosses, chains and shackles to the memory of the nameless, faceless, turfless Africans who met an untimely death in Faubourg Treme." The plaque goes on to say, "This St. Augustine/Treme shrine honors all slaves buried throughout the United States and those slaves in particular who lie beneath the ground of Treme in unmarked, unknown graves."

In 2008, the church was placed on the African American Heritage Trail for historic sites of cultural significance in Louisiana. You may arrange a tour by calling the church rectory at 504-525-5934. Mass, held every Sunday at 10 a.m., is yet another way to experience this historical landmark.

and parading traditions of the city's African American community. They include exhibits on Mardi Gras Indians, jazz funerals, social aid and pleasure clubs, Baby Dolls (female maskers in frilly attire), and Skull and Bone gangs, as well as filmed records of more than 500 events. In addition to hosting music and dance performances, conducting outreach programs, and creating an annual book that documents the year's jazz funerals, the museum serves as the starting and ending point for second-line parades and as an assembly spot for the North Side Skull and Bone Gang and Mardi Gras Indians on Fat Tuesday.

Walk a half block to Governor Nicholls Street, where at the intersection of Henriette Delille is ⑤ Sprouts Organic Cafe, a plant-based vegan restaurant. Turn left on Governor Nicholls. At the corner is ⑥ St. Augustine Catholic Church, the oldest African American Roman Catholic parish in the United States (see sidebar above).

Continue on Governor Nicholls, where at the corner of Treme Street, to your right, is the ⑦ Monrose Row Bed & Breakfast. The restored 1840s townhouse is one of many B&Bs in the neighborhood, catering to travelers who prefer the charm and quiet of Treme over the debauchery and loudness of the nearby French Quarter.

Just down Governor Nicholls from Monrose Row is the ⑧ New Orleans African American Museum of Art, Culture and History. Opened in 2000, its mission is "to preserve, interpret and promote the African American cultural heritage of New Orleans, with a particular emphasis on the Treme community." The museum offers walking tours covering such landmarks as St. Augustine Church, Congo Square, and a row of Creole cottages. Across the street is ⑨ Treme's Petit Jazz Museum, which is dedicated to the roots of jazz in Treme. If you're lucky, you'll get a personal tour from the owner Al Jackson, a jazz expert who achieved a life-long dream when he opened the museum in 2017.

Walk one block to North Robertson Street and turn left. ⑩ Fatma's Cozy Corner, a breakfast and lunch spot, is a block away at the intersection at Ursulines Avenue. From Fatma's, walk one and a half blocks to the ⑪ Candlelight Lounge, a legendary Treme music club. It's a dive, but a dive worth visiting, especially on Wednesday nights, when you can get free red beans and rice while enjoying the

*This famous archway welcomes visitors to experience the wonders of Louis Armstrong Park and Congo Square.*

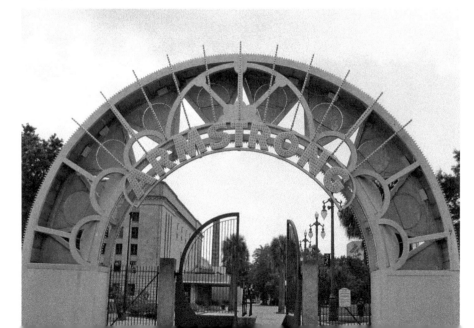

rollicking sounds of the Treme Brass Band. The band, led by snare drummer Benny Jones Sr., starts doing its thing around 9 p.m., and the place is almost always packed. Adjacent to the Candlelight is ⑫ Tuba Fats Square, named for Anthony "Tuba Fats" Lacen, a founding member of the Dirty Dozen Brass Band and, until his death in 2004, the city's most famous tuba player. Every year, on the Tuesday night after the New Orleans Jazz & Heritage Festival, some of the city's top brass musicians converge on Tuba Fats Square for Tuba Fats Tuesday, a musical celebration in Lacen's memory.

Though not on the walk, ⑬ Treme Coffeehouse, just down the block from Tuba Fats Square on St. Philip Street, provides a nice respite in between stops. You can choose from an array of coffee drinks, or if you prefer, ice cream or snowballs.

From Tuba Fats Square, walk two and a half blocks to Basin Street, cross Basin, and turn left. Circle right around Basin past the ⑭ Basin St. Station, a restored Southern Railway station that now serves as a visitor-information and cultural center. If you have time, stop in and learn about New Orleans through exhibits, murals, art, music, crafts, and entertainment.

Continue on Basin to St. Louis Street. At the corner is ⑮ St. Louis Cemetery No. 1. Founded in 1789 and listed on the National Register of Historic Places, it is the oldest existing cemetery in New Orleans. It's also the final resting spot for voodoo queen Marie Laveau; Étienne de Boré, the first mayor of New Orleans, who also produced the first granulated sugar; and Paul Morphy, a world-renowned chess player. If you're interested in walking through the cemetery, we strongly advise taking a formal tour. One of the best is conducted by Save Our Cemeteries, a nonprofit group dedicated to preserving the city's historic burial grounds. Ninety percent of the ticket price goes to cemetery restoration, education, and advocacy.

Cross Basin Street at St. Louis and walk one block to North Rampart Street. Turn left at North Rampart and continue back to the starting point at Louis Armstrong Park.

## Points of Interest

① Louis Armstrong Park  nola.gov/parks-and-parkways/parks-squares /congo-square-louis-armstrong-park, 701 N. Rampart St., 504-658-3200

② Bar Tonique  bartonique.com, 820 N. Rampart St., 504-324-6045

③ Effervescence  nolabubbles.com, 1036 N. Rampart St., 504-509-7644

④ Backstreet Cultural Museum  backstreetmuseum.org, 1116 Henriette Delille St., 504-522-4806

*(continued on next page)*

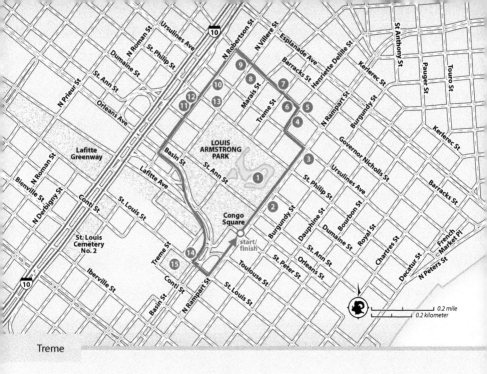

Treme

(continued from previous page)

⑤ Sprouts Organic Cafe  sproutsorganiccafe.com, 1200 Henriette Delille St., 504-919-1221

⑥ St. Augustine Catholic Church  staugchurch.org, 1210 Governor Nicholls St., 504-525-5934

⑦ Monrose Row Bed & Breakfast  monroserow.com, 1303 Governor Nicholls St., 504-616-6377

⑧ African American Museum of Art, Culture and History  noaam.org, 1418 Governor Nicholls St., 504-566-1136

⑨ Treme's Petit Jazz Museum  tremespetitjazzmuseum.com, 1500 Governor Nicholls St., 504-715-0332

⑩ Fatma's Cozy Corner  facebook.com/19parkisland, 1532 Ursulines Ave., 504-708-5896

⑪ Candlelight Lounge  facebook.com/Candlelightlounge925/, 925 N. Robertson St., 504-525-4748

⑫ Tuba Fats Square  1600 St. Philip St.

⑬ Treme Coffeehouse  thetremecoffeehouse.com, 1505 St. Philip St., 504-218-8663

⑭ Basin St. Station  basinststation.com, 501 Basin St., 504-293-2600

⑮ St. Louis Cemetery No. 1  saveourcemeteries.org, 320 N. Claiborne Ave., 504-596-3050

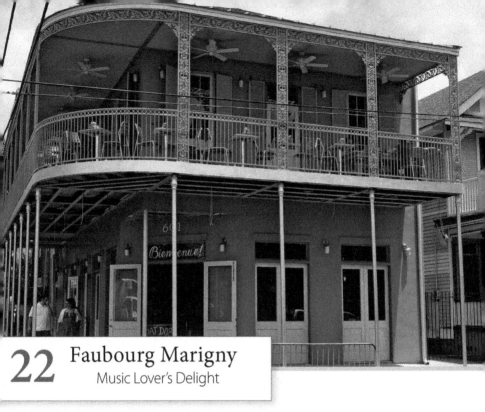

# 22 Faubourg Marigny
## Music Lover's Delight

*Above: Dat Dog is a great place to grab a gourmet frank while club-hopping.*
photo by Donna Goldenberg

BOUNDARIES: Elysian Fields Ave., Esplanade Ave., Dauphine St., N. Peters St.
DISTANCE: 1.54 miles
PARKING: Metered parking, parking lots, some free street parking
PUBLIC TRANSIT: Riverfront Streetcar

Ask local music lovers where they enjoy listening to jazz, blues, rock, and funk, and you're sure to hear names like Tipitina's in Uptown, Howlin' Wolf in the Warehouse District, and the Rock'n'Bowl in Carrollton. You may also hear names like Snug Harbor, Blue Nile, and Spotted Cat, three of a bounty of clubs that make up the fun, funky music scene on Frenchmen Street in historic Faubourg Marigny.

The people you ask may or may not share those details, however: locals tend to want to keep the Marigny—as it's commonly called—to themselves, though even they recognize that it's becoming a hot spot for tourists, particularly those looking for fun off the beaten path.

Just downriver of the French Quarter, the Marigny (MARE-uh-nee) is one of the coolest, most eclectic neighborhoods in all of New Orleans, and that's saying a lot, considering the uniqueness of each one. On Frenchmen Street, the main drag, you'll find tattoo parlors, art galleries, restaurants, a bike shop, and, the biggest draw of all, music clubs. It's a popular "Hollywood South" locale as well, with the TV crime drama *NCIS: New Orleans* and the 2014 flick *Chef* among productions that have shot here.

But Faubourg Marigny is far more than an entertainment district. It has an equally fascinating history, its development going back to 1805 when millionaire developer Bernard de Marigny (who popularized the game of craps) subdivided his family's plantation to create what is considered New Orleans's first suburb. Although the neighborhood began to deteriorate in the 1950s, renewed interest in its history, culture, and architecture led to its rebirth in the early 1970s, when it was placed on the National Register of Historic Places. Today, the Marigny is thriving, with beautifully restored Victorian shotguns and Creole cottages, many painted in eye-popping colors, lining the streets.

## Walk Description

Begin at Elysian Fields Avenue and Dauphine Street, in front of ❶ Washington Square, a 2.5-acre park that serves as a popular hangout for residents and venue for festivals, art markets, and other events. One of the highlights of the square is the New Orleans AIDS Memorial, a series of glass discs depicting the faces of AIDS in the city.

Walk four blocks to North Peters Street. Circle right to Esplanade Avenue in front of ❷ Hotel de la Monnaie, a European-style timeshare property on the edge of the French Quarter. Just next door is the ❸ Dragon's Den, the first of many music clubs you'll encounter as you veer right onto Frenchmen Street, one of the city's most popular music districts. Over the next three blocks, you'll pass ❹ the Yard on Frenchmen, a patio garden bar and eatery; ❺ Louisiana Music Factory, a music store that occasionally hosts free concerts; ❻ Vaso, a so-called ultralounge with brass bands, DJs, and food; and ❼ the Maison, a live-music venue that boasts three levels and three stages.

Other clubs on Frenchmen include ❽ Bamboula's, which combines the blues with Caribbean cuisine; ❾ 13 Monaghan, where the specialty menu item is Tater Tot nachos ("Tachos"); and ❿ Blue Nile, which stages funk, blues, soul, and brass-band shows in a building dating back to 1832. ⓫ Three Muses is a restaurant and music club where you can munch on such fare as Gulf fish tacos, braised meatballs, or blue cheese–stuffed dates while taking in the sounds of singer and trombonist Glen David Andrews or pianist Tom McDermott. ⓬ Favela Chic got its start as a taco truck and prides itself on casual but oh-so-tasty Latin American fare.

Cross Chartres Street and continue down Frenchmen past more attractions, including ⑬ Frenchmen Art and Books, which has delighted book lovers since 1978. You'll also pass more more clubs and restaurants, including ⑭ Dat Dog, famous for its gourmet hot dogs and sausages; ⑮ Cafe Negril, a reggae club that shares space with a po'boy joint called ⑯ Po-Breaux's; ⑰ Spotted Cat, known for its old-time swing jazz; and ⑱ d.b.a., where regular performers include some of the hottest names in New Orleans music, among them Walter "Wolfman" Washington, Jon Cleary, the Soul Rebels, and the Treme Brass Band. At the legendary ⑲ Snug Harbor, contemporary jazz greats Charmaine Neville, Donald Harrison, and the Uptown Jazz Orchestra pack in the crowds. And at the corner of Frenchmen and Royal, ⑳ Marigny Brasserie serves up a menu of Creole cuisine along with such entertainers as the Pfister Sisters, Paul Sanchez, and the Washboard Chaz Blues Trio. ㉑ Apple Barrel rounds out the medley of music clubs. ㉒ Adolfo's, on the second floor of Apple Barrel, is a Creole-Italian eatery whose signature dish is corn-and-crab cannelloni. If you're visiting Frenchmen on Thursday through Sunday nights, stop by the ㉓ Palace Market Frenchmen, an art market in the lot next to Spotted Cat.

*Spotted Cat Music Club calls itself the "quintessential jazz club" of New Orleans.*
photo by Donna Goldenberg

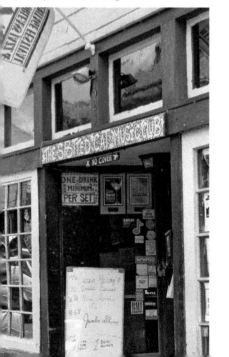

Turn left on Royal Street and walk one block to the intersection of Royal and Touro Street. Continue down Royal, cross Kerlerec Street, walk another block to Esplanade Avenue, and turn right. This is a mostly residential area, but a number of bed-and-breakfasts and guest houses line this stretch. Among them is the Royal Street Inn (1431 Royal), home of the hopping ㉔ R Bar, a dive that draws huge crowds for its affordable drinks and funky vibe. For *NCIS: New Orleans* fans, it's better known as the Tru Tone Bar, one of Agent Pride's favorite hangouts.

Cross Esplanade at Dauphine Street, turn left, and begin walking back down Esplanade to the starting point. Don't be surprised to see a crowd of people standing in front of 838 Esplanade. This is ㉕ Port of Call, which, even with the proliferation of burger restaurants around town, is still considered one of the city's best.

# The New Orleans Jazz Museum

In a neighborhood brimming with music clubs, there might not be a better place to learn about the history of jazz—and listen to it—than the New Orleans Jazz Museum, one of 12 sites that make up the Louisiana State Museum.

Formerly the Old US Mint, the building was once used to mint both Union and Confederate currency. The Greek Revival–style structure became a museum in 1981, boasting such permanent exhibits as "New Orleans Jazz," which features instruments, sheet music, and memorabilia depicting the history of the genre in New Orleans, along with a photography gallery showcasing some of the city's premier musicians.

Today, the museum offers a series of five rotating exhibits related to jazz history and culture, including exhibits on drumming, legendary jazz musicians Louis Prima and Professor Longhair, and the music photography of Rick Olivier. Each exhibit features listening stations, films, and instruments. The third floor performance center offers live music, theatrical performances, lectures, symposia oral histories, and panel discussions.

You'll pass several Victorian mansions on both sides of Esplanade, including the ㉖ Lanaux Mansion (to your left at 547 Esplanade), an 1879 Renaissance Revival home that *Forbes* magazine has called one of the best bed-and-breakfasts in the country. The exterior of the inn and its lobby were featured in the Brad Pitt film *The Curious Case of Benjamin Button*. The inn's decor includes original furniture and wallpapers from 1879, as well as Civil War memorabilia. Registered guests can arrange for a tour upon their arrival.

Music venues abound on this stretch as well, among them ㉗ Igor's Checkpoint Charlie (501 Esplanade Ave.), which specializes in alternative-rock and metal bands, and the ㉘ Balcony Music Club (BMC), at the corner of Esplanade and Decatur Street, which features blues, funk, and R&B bands.

From BMC, cross Decatur and you'll be in front of the ㉙ New Orleans Jazz Museum, one of several museums that make up the Louisiana State Museum (see sidebar above). Built in 1835, the Greek Revival building served as a branch of the U.S. Mint for both the Union and the Confederacy. Today, it's home to exhibits, complete with listening stations and films, on such New Orleans jazz greats as Professor Longhair, Louis Prima, and more.

Cross Esplanade at North Peters Street, then circle left on North Peters, which becomes Elysian Fields Avenue heading north. Cross on Elysian Fields where North Peters picks up again heading right, but be cautious, as this is an especially busy intersection.

Continue down North Peters one block to Marigny Street and turn left. Tucked in this mostly residential neighborhood are restaurants like ㉚ Paladar 511, watering holes like ㉛ The Friendly

Bar, and just off Marigny on Burgundy Street, **㉜ Hotel Peter and Paul.** The hotel is the result of a four-year restoration of the old St. Peter and Paul church, school house, convent, and rectory. In addition to more than 70 rooms, the hotel is home to **㉝ The Elysian** bar, café, and patio and **㉞ Sundae Best**, which specializes in handcrafted ice cream made with locally sourced ingredients.

Turn left on Burgundy and walk one block to Elysian Fields. Cross Elysian Fields, turn left, and walk one block back to Washington Square.

*No two rooms are alike at Hotel Peter and Paul.*

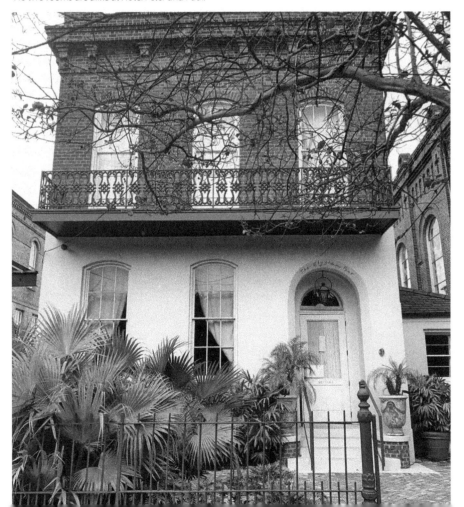

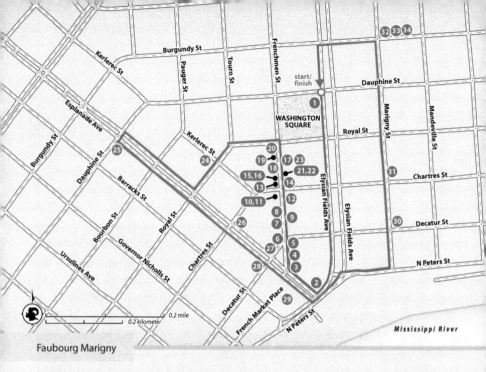

Faubourg Marigny

## Points of Interest

1. Washington Square  nola.gov/parks-and-parkways/parks-squares/washington-square, bounded by Elysian Fields Avenue and Frenchmen, Dauphine, and Royal Streets; 504-658-3200

2. Hotel de la Monnaie  hoteldelamonnaie.com, 405 Esplanade Ave., 504-947-0009

3. Dragon's Den  dragonsdennola.com, 435 Esplanade Ave.

4. The Yard on Frenchmen  theyardneworleans.com, 405 Frenchmen St., 504-266-2848

5. Louisiana Music Factory  louisianamusicfactory.com, 421 Frenchmen St., 504-586-1094

6. Vaso  facebook.com/vasonola, 500 Frenchmen St., 504-272-0929

7. The Maison  maisonfrenchmen.com, 508 Frenchmen St., 504-371-5543

8. Bamboula's  bamboulasnola.com, 514 Frenchmen St., 504-944-8461

9. 13 Monaghan  13monaghan.com, 517 Frenchmen St., 504-942-1345

10. Blue Nile  bluenilelive.com, 532 Frenchmen St., 504-948-2583

11. Three Muses  3musesnola.com, 536 Frenchmen St., 504-252-4801

12. Favela Chic  favelachicnola.com, 525 Frenchmen St., 504-400-3930

13. Frenchmen Art and Books  frenchmenartandbooks.com, 600 Frenchmen St., 504-302-1772

⑭ Dat Dog  datdognola.com, 601 Frenchmen St., 504-309-3362

⑮ Cafe Negril  cafenegrilonfrenchmen.com, 606 Frenchmen St., 504-229-4236

⑯ Po-Breaux's  pobreauxs.com, 606 Frenchmen St., 504-229-4236

⑰ Spotted Cat  spottedcatmusicclub.com, 623 Frenchmen St., 504-943-3887

⑱ d.b.a.  dbaneworleans.com, 618 Frenchmen St., 504-942-3731

⑲ Snug Harbor  snugjazz.com, 626 Frenchmen St., 504-949-0696

⑳ Marigny Brasserie  marignybrasserie.com, 640 Frenchmen St., 504-945-4472

㉑ Apple Barrel  tinyurl.com/applebarrelnola, 609 Frenchmen St., 504-949-9399

㉒ Adolfo's  tinyurl.com/adolfosnola, 611 Frenchmen St., 504-948-3800

㉓ Palace Market Frenchmen  palacemarketnola.com, 619 Frenchmen St., 504-358-8287

㉔ R Bar  royalstreetinn.com/r-bar, 1431 Royal St., 504-948-7499

㉕ Port of Call  portofcallnola.com, 838 Esplanade Ave., 504-523-0120

㉖ Lanaux Mansion Bed and Breakfast  lanauxmansion.com, 547 Esplanade Ave., 504-330-2826

㉗ Igor's Checkpoint Charlie  501 Esplanade Ave., 504-281-4847

㉘ Balcony Music Club  balconymusicclub.com, 1331 Decatur St., 504-301-5912

㉙ New Orleans Jazz Museum (formerly the Old US Mint)  nolajazzmuseum.org, 400 Esplanade Ave., 504-568-6993

㉚ Paladar 511  paladar511.com, 511 Marigny St., 504-509-6782

㉛ The Friendly Bar  2301 Chartres St., 504-943-8929

㉜ Hotel Peter and Paul  hotelpeterandpaul.com, 2317 Burgundy St., 504-356-5200

㉝ The Elysian  theelysianbar.com, 2317 Burgundy St., 504-356-6769

㉞ Sundae Best  sundaebesticecream.com, 2317 Burgundy St., 504-656-4746

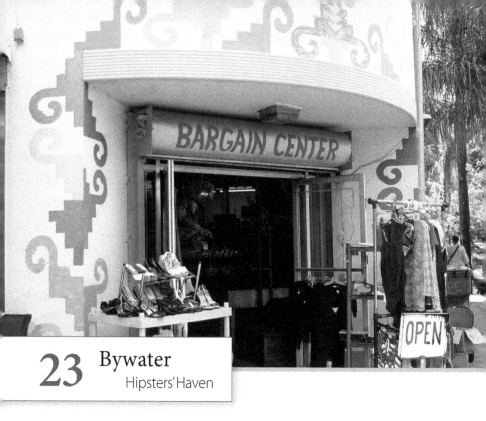

# 23 Bywater
## Hipsters' Haven

*Above: The Bargain Center thrift store is a perfect fit for this bohemian neighborhood.*

BOUNDARIES: St. Claude Ave., Chartres St., Piety St., Montegut St.
DISTANCE: 1.29 miles
PARKING: Free street parking
PUBLIC TRANSIT: RTA Bus #5 (Marigny-Bywater)

A lot of words have been tossed about to describe the Bywater section of New Orleans, and, well, most of them are true. The neighborhood along the Mississippi River between Faubourg Marigny and the Industrial Canal is perhaps the funkiest, edgiest, most bohemian 'hood in New Orleans. And yeah, we may as well throw in the term *hipster* too.

The evolution of Bywater as the city's "it" neighborhood began after Hurricane Katrina in 2005, and it has been exploding in popularity ever since. Because of its higher elevation along the river, it escaped the flooding that destroyed so many other parts of town. As a result, the so-called "Sliver by the River" became a magnet for folks looking for new places to lay roots. Of late, Bywater has become a haven for newcomers, along with artists and musicians.

The houses alone make this neighborhood something special. We're not talking mansions—we're talking Creole cottages and shotgun doubles painted in eye-popping shades of purple, orange, and blue, and trimmed in equally vibrant colors. The houses are so much fun to look at that one could easily miss everything else this neighborhood has to offer, from restaurants and music clubs to arts venues and parks, including Crescent Park, a 1.4-mile linear park built along the river.

## Walk Description

Start your walk at the intersection of Chartres Street and Homer Plessy Way, right in front of the ❶ New Orleans Center for Creative Arts, also known as NOCCA, a creative arts high school whose famous alumni include Harry Connick Jr., Wynton and Branford Marsalis, Terence Blanchard, Wendell Pierce, and Anthony Mackie. The school offers training in music, visual arts, jazz, dance, culinary arts, creative writing, musical theater, drama, and more. From NOCCA, continue on Chartres a half block past ❷ Bywater American Bistro, whose chef-owner is Nina Compton of *Top Chef: New Orleans* fame. The restaurant, located on the first floor of the Rice Mill Lofts, is considered the gateway to the Bywater.

Continue walking down Chartres Street, where at 3027 Chartres you'll pass ❸ Dr. Bob's Folk Art, the sign shop of renowned New Orleans artist Bob Shaffer. Dr. Bob has sold his colorful and funky folk art worldwide, and is best known for his visual message BE NICE OR LEAVE. If you drop in for a visit, you may just see Dr. Bob at work creating one of his signature cityscapes, shotgun houses, or gators, most featuring found objects like bottle caps and reclaimed wood.

Turn left on Clouet Street and walk two blocks to Dauphine Street. On the way, you'll pass ❹ Bureau of Change, a collaborative digital media studio where artists create, curate, and exhibit socially and politically engaged work; ❺ Petite Clouet Café, a friendly lunch and breakfast spot; and ❻ Clouet Gardens, a neighborhood park.

At the corner of Clouet and Dauphine, look at the church to your left. The church is home of the ❼ Blessed Francis Xavier Seelos Catholic Church. Listed on the National Register of Historic Places, the church opened in 1838 as St. Vincent de Paul Parish but was renamed in 2001 for Seelos, a Redemptorist priest known for his devotion to the poor and abandoned. Two years later, the interior of the church was destroyed by a fire but has since been restored. The church has stunning stained glass windows and a massive pipe organ donated by a group of Seattle-based churches whose volunteers had come to New Orleans to help in the Katrina recovery. The church is also home to the St. Gerard Community for the Deaf, which serves the spiritual needs of the area's deaf and hearing-impaired Catholics.

Turn right on Dauphine and walk two blocks to the corner of Dauphine and Louisa Streets. On your stroll, take note of the sheer variety of houses, among them 19th- and 20th-century shotgun doubles, Creole cottages, and Craftsman bungalows, many of which have been transformed from dilapidated shacks to architectural masterpieces.

At the corner of Dauphine and Louisa, to your left, is ⑧ Alma Cafe, a modern Honduran eatery that specializes in such fare as salsa verde ceviche, homemade chicharróns (cracklins), and *guiso* (stew).

A neighborhood like Bywater needs a good thrift store, so if you're in the market for second-hand stuff, check out the ⑨ Bargain Center, at the opposite corner of Dauphine and Louisa. The place is packed to the gills with everything from antiques and jewelry to vintage photographs and Mexican folk art.

Continue walking in the 3200 block of Dauphine. At 3218 Dauphine is ⑩ Satsuma Cafe, a cool eatery with an especially impressive selection of fresh-squeezed organic juices, from the Popeye (a mixture of spinach, lemon, kale, and apple) to the Cleanser (beet, fennel, cucumber, and lemon). The quinoa salad and the roasted-pear-and-brie melt are among the yummy items on the menu.

At the end of the block on the left, at the corner of Dauphine and Piety, is ⑪ Frady's One Stop Food Store, a convenience store that also makes a pretty decent po'boy, perfect for matching with a cold beer and enjoying at one of the outdoor tables.

Turn right on Piety Street and walk one block to Royal Street past ⑫ Mickey Markey Park, once a rundown playground that received a much-needed upgrade when city officials shut it down several years ago because of high levels of lead contamination. In addition to remediation work, the park received fresh landscaping, updated playground equipment, and new concrete walkways.

Walk one block to Chartres Street past ⑬ Pizza Delicious, which got its start as a twice-a-week pop-up. It proved so popular that when the owners decided to open a permanent eatery on Piety, they were able to raise some of their startup money through crowd sourcing. Pizza Delicious serves traditional New York–style pizza like cheese and pepperoni but also offers a special pizza of the day. Past pizza specials have included braised Brussels sprouts, wild boar and charred green onion sausage, and roasted cauliflower and marinated red onion. Pizza Delicious has made two national best-of lists: its Hot Sopressata was named one of the website Thrillist's "Top 33 Pizzas in America," and its plain cheese pizza was honored as one of the Daily Meal's "101 Best Pizzas in America."

Next door to Pizza Delicious is ⑭ Bratz Y'all, a traditional German beer garden specializing in bratwurst, schnitzel, and other German fare. Across the street is the Old Ironworks, which hosts

# Crescent Park

It was eight years in the making, but when Crescent Park opened in February 2014 along the Mississippi River, it was hailed as a major step in the city's revitalization. City officials said it also fulfilled their mission of returning the riverfront to the people.

Stretching from Bywater to the Marigny, the 20-acre linear park is located at what was once a thriving wharf area, and its design and layout are in keeping with its industrial past. The park features 20 acres of indigenous landscaping, bike paths, playgrounds, a dog run, and the first of two multiuse pavilions transformed from former industrial wharves, including the Piety Wharf, which overlooks the Mississippi River and the New Orleans skyline and includes a garden and picnic area. One of the park's signature features is the Piety Street Arch, a pedestrian footbridge that crosses active railroad tracks and the Mississippi River floodwall. The Mandeville Shed is an old industrial wharf that has been converted into an open-air event space, and the Mandeville Ellipse is a raised grass lawn popular for weddings and corporate events. The park offers a variety of community activities, from yoga to dance classes.

Park hours are 6 a.m.–7:30 p.m. A public parking lot is located along Chartres Street at the foot of Piety Street.

monthly flea markets, theatrical productions, festivals, and other events. Next to Bratz Y'all, in the hot-pink building at the corner of Piety and Chartres, is ⓯ Euclid Records, which, in addition to selling new and used vinyl and CDs, stages live-music performances.

Turn right on Chartres. Across the street is an arched staircase leading across railroad tracks to ⓰ Crescent Park, a 1.4-mile linear green space that stretches from Elysian Fields Avenue in the Marigny to Mazant Street in Bywater (see sidebar above). The park isn't included on this tour but is highly recommended.

Walk one block and turn right on Louisa Street. Toward the end of the block, at 634 Louisa, is one of Bywater's most elegant homes, a late-19th-century raised center-hall Italianate cottage. This is home to the ⓱ Country Club, which has a restaurant and bar inside and a swimming pool, cabana bar, and hot tub out back (the backyard amenities cost extra).

In contrast to the stateliness of the Country Club is its next-door neighbor, ⓲ Markey's Bar, a congenial dive that's been open since 1947. Markey's is a popular gathering spot for watching sports or trying one or two of the 25 beers on tap.

Turn left at Markey's onto Royal Street and walk three blocks to Homer Plessy Way. Along this stretch you'll pass ⓳ The Tigermen Den, an event space housed in a 19th-century Creole corner store. The place is named for the all-female band the Tigermen, who once lived in an upstairs apartment and used the first floor for rehearsals. Among the events held at the Den are monthly Cajun brunches where you can learn the Cajun two-step, weekly jazz nights, yoga classes, and art exhibitions.

In the next block, at the corner of Royal and Montegut Streets is ⑳ **The London Clayworks**, a ceramic studio that caters to professionals and amateurs alike. In the next block, you'll pass ㉑ **Studio Be**, the art studio of New Orleans filmmaker and visual artist Brendan "BMike" Odums. The 36,000-square-foot gallery features wall-size murals and installations that largely reflect the political passion of today's Black activism. The studio is open to the public four days a week.

Continue down Royal to the intersection of Homer Plessy Way. To the right is the ㉒ *Plessy vs. Ferguson Historical Marker*, which marks the spot where Plessy, a free person of color, was tossed off a railway car and arrested in 1892. Plessy had defied a Louisiana law that segregated railroad trains on the basis of race, and his law-suit against the state of Louisiana (and Judge Howard Ferguson) made it all the way to the US Supreme Court. Although the high court held the Louisiana segregation statute constitutional, the case is commonly considered the beginning of the civil rights movement.

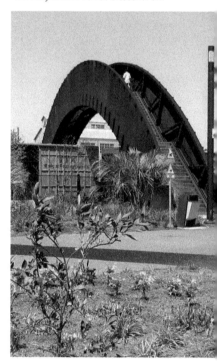

*The Piety Street Arch at Crescent Park*

Across Royal at the intersection of Homer Plessy Way is ㉓ **Press Street Station**, a project of the NOCCA Institute, the nonprofit arm of the New Orleans Center for Creative Arts. The restored railway facility and warehouse is a special-events venue, with proceeds from rentals supporting NOCCA students and faculty.

Continue down Royal past ㉔ JAMNOLA, which stands for Joy, Art, Music—New Orleans. The 54,000-square-foot experience takes audiences of all ages on a stroll through the cultural gems that make the Crescent City the unique place that it is. JAMNOLA is the brainchild of two Bywater residents, Chad Smith and Jonny Liss, who teamed up with the nonprofit Where Y'art to create 12 interactive exhibits celebrating the city's art, music, food, and theatrics through the eyes of 20 local artists. A portion of the proceeds from JAMNOLA is donated to charity partners Trombone Shorty Foundation and Feed the Second Line.

Walk down Homer Plessey Way one block to the starting point. As you make your way back to NOCCA, consider a stop at the ㉕ 5 Press Gallery, which features the artwork of NOCCA alumni and faculty.

Although this is the end of the tour, there is so much more to Bywater, and we'd be remiss in not mentioning the neighborhood's other treasures—Bywater Bakery (3624 Dauphine St.), known for some of the best pastries in town; Elizabeth's (601 Gallier St.), a down-home restaurant famous for its praline bacon and fried green tomatoes; the music clubs Vaughn's Lounge (4229 Dauphine St.) and B. J.'s Lounge (4301 Burgundy St); and Bacchanal (600 Poland Ave.), a wine bar with a cool outdoor patio. For barbecue, try the Joint (701 Mazant St.); for fried seafood, Jack Dempsey's (738 Poland Ave.).

## Points of Interest

① New Orleans Center for Creative Arts  nocca.com, 2800 Chartres St., 504-940-2787

② Bywater American Bistro  bywateramericanbistro.com, 2900 Chartres St., 504-605-3827

③ Dr. Bob's Folk Art  drbobart.net, 3027 Chartres St., 504-945-2225

④ Bureau of Change  bureauofchange.org, 638 Clouet St.

⑤ Petite Clouet Café  facebook.com/petiteclouet, 3100 Royal St.

⑥ Clouet Gardens  710 Clouet St., 504-234-9545

⑦ Blessed Francis Xavier Seelos Catholic Church  seeloschurchno.org, 3053 Dauphine St., 504-943-5566

⑧ Alma Cafe  eatalmanola.com, 800 Louisa St., 504-381-5877

⑨ Bargain Center  3200 Dauphine St., 504-948-0007

⑩ Satsuma Cafe  satsumacafe.com, 3218 Dauphine St., 504-304-5962

⑪ Frady's One Stop Food Store  3231 Dauphine St., 504-949-9688

⑫ Mickey Markey Park  700 Piety St.

⑬ Pizza Delicious  pizzadelicious.com, 617 Piety St., 504-676-8482

⑭ Bratz Y'all  bratzyall.com, 617-B Piety St., 504-301-3222

⑮ Euclid Records  euclidrecordsneworleans.com, 3301 Chartres St., 504-947-4348

*(continued on next page)*

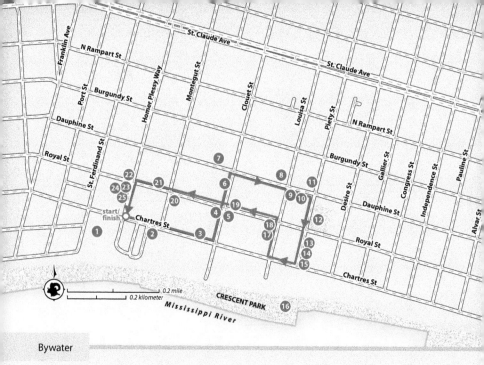

Bywater

(continued from previous page)

16. Crescent Park  crescentparknola.org, Mississippi Riverfront between Elysian Fields Ave. and Mazant St., 504-658-4334

17. The Country Club  thecountryclubneworleans.com, 634 Louisa St., 504-945-0742

18. Markey's Bar  facebook.com/markeysbarnola, 640 Louisa St., 504-943-0785

19. The Tigermen Den  thetigermenden.com, 3113 Royal St., 504-230-0131

20. The London Clayworks  thelondonclayworks.com, 3000 Royal St., 504-313-8506

21. Studio Be  bmike.com, 2941 Royal St., 504-252-0463

22. *Plessy vs. Ferguson Historical Marker*  700 Homer Plessy Way

23. Press Street Station  pressstreetstation.com, 5 Homer Plessy Way, 504-940-2986

24. JAMNOLA  jamnola.com, 2832 Royal St., 504-233-9152

25. 5 Press Gallery  noccainstitute.com, 5 Homer Plessy Way, 504-940-2986

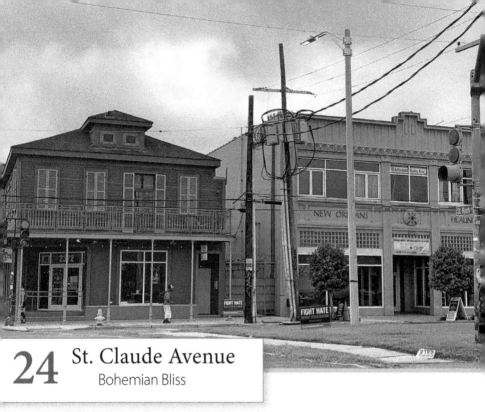

# 24 St. Claude Avenue
## Bohemian Bliss

---

*Above: Buildings painted in bold colors are typical of the St. Claude Avenue neighborhood.*

---

BOUNDARIES: Elysian Fields Avenue, St. Claude Avenue, Desire Street
DISTANCE: 2.02 miles
PARKING: Street parking
PUBLIC TRANSIT: RTA Bus #5 (Marigny-Bywater)

---

It's no St. Charles Avenue, that's for sure. You won't find stately mansions on St. Claude Avenue, nor will you find canopies of oak trees, historic churches, or luxury salons and boutiques.

But what you will find on this gritty, colorful thoroughfare in the Upper Ninth Ward is, in many ways, just as appealing. In addition to iconic places such as Capt. Sal's Seafood and Chicken and the Hi-Ho Lounge, which have been around for decades, you'll find art galleries and performing arts venues, tattoo parlors and vaping shops, vintage clothing stores and coffeehouses.

You'll spot bold, edgy, and thought-provoking street art almost everywhere you look. And you'll encounter some of the most fascinating and acclaimed restaurants in the city. In fact, the travel guide *Frommer's* called St. Claude "the next big thing in great food."

Although the neighborhood began attracting artists in the late 1990s, it wasn't until after Hurricane Katrina that St. Claude—one of the few areas that didn't flood in the storm—began to emerge as a full-fledged arts district. The culinary component soon followed, making St. Claude a destination for tourists and locals alike. If you plan to take either the Bywater or Marigny tours included in this book, you might want to add St. Claude to your walk. As you'll soon discover, there are lots of places on the route to take a break and enjoy the colorful people and places that make St. Claude the unique street that it is.

## Walk Description

Begin this walk at the ❶ St. Roch Market, a sleek, white-pillared food hall that occupies space that served as an open-air market in the 19th century and more recently a seafood market. St. Roch features more than a dozen vendors representing an array of cultures, from Mexican to Malaysian. Elysian Seafood and Oyster Bar specializes in raw and chargrilled oysters, Louisiana crab cakes, and blackened shrimp po'boys. And the Mayhaw is a cocktail bar that promises a "specially curated experience that celebrates quality, craftsmanship and creativity."

Facing St. Claude at St. Roch Market, turn left and walk three blocks to St. Claude and Port Street. Cross Port Street at the ❷ Maypop Community Herb Shop, which works to serve as a community resource for plant knowledge, remedies, healing, and social change. It specializes in medicinal herbs, culinary spices, and teas along with soaps, salves, oils, lotions, incenses, and essential oils.

Walk one block and cross St. Ferdinand Street. On this block you'll pass ❸ Gerken's Bike Shop, ❹ Poke-Chan, and ❺ Faubourg Wines, the latter of which sells wines from around the world, along with artisanal cheeses and meats, chocolates, olive oils, mustards, and wine vinegars. If you have time, grab a seat at the bar and let the owners recommend a glass of wine that fits your style and budget.

Walk three blocks to Montegut Street. Just down the block on Montegut is ❻ N7, a French restaurant and wine bar founded by filmmaker Aaron Walker and chef Yuki Yamaguchi. The name of the restaurant is derived from Nationale 7 (N7), the highway that once ran from Paris to the border of Italy. The highway was commonly known as Route des Vacances because so many Parisians used it to travel south on vacation. According to the folks at N7, it was such a popular route that the *Michelin Guide* would direct travelers to the mom-and-pop restaurants housed in farmhouses and hotels. N7 specializes in French cuisine, often with a Japanese flair—sake-cured salmon tartine, escargot tempura, and soy sauce crème brûlée are some of the dishes on the menu.

Continue walking down St. Claude past the **7** **Junction Bar & Grill**, a tavern that offers 40 beers on tap and an impressive selection of creative Boxcar Burgers, along with salads, wings, and snacks. At the corner of Clouet Street and St. Claude, about a block away, is the **Saturn Bar**, a legendary dive known for cheap drinks, live music, and dance parties. As of this writing, Saturn had closed, but a pending sale was in the works, with plans to keep the property as a bar.

Walk three blocks to Desire Street, just past another funky joint called **8** **Stuph'D Beignets and Burgers**, where, in addition to traditional sugar-laden beignets, you can get beignets stuffed with any number of sweet or savory fillings. One such beignet is the Creole Queen, stuffed with crawfish, crabmeat, and shrimp.

Cross St. Claude at Desire, turn right, and make your way down the opposite side of the avenue. On the first block, you'll pass **9** **Rosalita's Backyard Tacos**, which got its start in the owners' back-yard in Bywater and became so popular that the couple, Ian Schnoebelen and Laurie Casebonne, opened a real restaurant, complete with a backyard. Specialty fare includes such tacos as pork belly, al pastor, fried fish, and smoked pork and brisket.

Walk a block to Piety Street. Just down Piety to your left is **10** **Robert Emery Chocolate**, a choc-olate lover's paradise that sells 80 flavors of hand-rolled and hand-dipped chocolates, both toffees and truffles. (At press time, the shop was operating online only due to the COVID-19 pandemic.)

Walk another block to Louisa Street, where at the corner to your left is a neighborhood institution—**11** **Capt. Sal's Seafood and Chicken**. If you're in the market for traditional Creole- and Cajun-influenced seafood dishes, be it crawfish, gumbo, jambalaya, or crab, all made with a secret batter recipe that the chef promises has the perfect amount of spiciness, this is the place to try. Also in this block is **12** **Art Space 3116**, a gallery and private event venue that regularly holds art exhibitions, musical performances, and other arts events.

Continue walking down St. Claude to the block between Clouet and Montegut Streets. This block alone is a culinary haven, with a plethora of restaurants, both upscale and casual, from which to choose. There's **13** **Galaxie**, **14** **Saint-Germain**, and **15** **Red's Chinese** among them. Galaxie is a highly acclaimed taqueria housed in an old Texaco gas station that is listed on the National Register of Historic Places. Saint-Germain is a tiny French restaurant—the dining room has only 12 seats—where guests experience a five-course tasting menu. Reservations are a must, but if you can't get in, feel free to drop in at the wine bar, which offers an extensive selection of wine, beer, and cocktails, along with snacks like pâté and fresh cheese with country bread. Red's Chinese has built a reputation for having some of the best Asian fare in the city. Dishes include kung pao pastrami, crawfish Rangoon, and ginger scallion noodle. Also on this block is ⑯ The Domino, a wine bar that hosts pop-ups, trivia nights, and tabletop games; ⑰ The Grand Maltese, an art gallery; and ⑱ The Get Down NOLA, a live-music club.

Walk three blocks to Port Street. On this stretch, you'll pass ⑲ St. Coffee, a combination coffee bar and snowball stand, and ⑳ The New Movement, a comedy theater featuring improv, stand-up, and sketch shows, along with improv classes for children and adults.

Continue walking down St. Claude to Franklin Avenue, a major intersection. To your left on Franklin is ㉑ Chakras NOLA, a vintage clothing store that also sells costumes and local art. Just down the block, on St. Claude, is the ㉒ Artisan Bar & Cafe, where owners Dave Grove and Dave Stewart pride themselves not just on their menu but also on the atmosphere. They describe their café as a "happy, healthy, safe and inclusive space that is welcoming to all people. There are no strangers, just friends we haven't met."

Walk another block to the intersection of St. Claude and Music Streets. ㉓ Morrow's, at the corner, is another NOLA restaurant that has received high praise from critics and locals alike. In fact, *The New York Times* included it on a list of "Five Places to Visit in New Orleans." Morrow's is described by its owners, Chef Lenora Chong and her son Larry Morrow, as a place "where great food and dope vibes collide." The menu combines Korean fare with New Orleans cuisine. At the end of the block, at St. Roch Avenue, ㉔ Byrdie's Pottery is a nonprofit ceramics studio that offers classes as well as space for creating and selling pottery.

The next block, between St. Roch and Spain Streets, is another one of those blocks that is chock-full of places to visit. Among them is the ㉕ New Orleans Healing Center, a community center that operates under the United Nations guidelines for sustainability. As such, it offers services that aim to help, heal, and empower individuals and the neighborhood at the economic, social, environmental, physical, mental, and spiritual levels. The center houses a yoga studio, a food co-op, a dance studio, a physical therapy center, an animal health clinic, and healing arts services, such as acupuncture, massage therapy, and hypnotherapy. There's even a space called the Free Little Pantry, which stocks food, toiletries, and other goods for families in need. Its motto: "Take what you need, leave what you can." Also housed at the Healing Center, in the back on St. Roch and N. Rampart Streets, is ㉖ Café Istanbul, an entertainment venue that showcases music, theater, dance, and comedy acts. It also has an art gallery, where it displays the work of local painters and photographers on a monthly rotating basis.

Down the block from the Healing Center are the ㉗ New Orleans Boulder Lounge, a rock-climbing venue, and ㉘ Vintage Voyage, which sells clothing, costumes, and curiosities.

Walk three blocks to Elysian Fields Avenue, past ㉙ Bao and Noodle, a casual Chinese eatery; ㉚ Arabella Casa di Pasta, known for build-your-own pasta bowls; ㉛ AllWays Lounge and Cabaret, which stages burlesque, comedy, and theatrical performances; and ㉜ Nola Mia, which, in addition to gelato and other amazing desserts, specializes in pizza and paninis.

Just to the left of the corner of St. Claude and Elysian Fields is ㉝ Baldwin & Co. bookshop, which features books of almost every genre, as well as a café offering an array of coffees, teas, and pastries. Feel free to head that way before you begin your walk back to the starting point.

Cross St. Claude at Elysian Fields, turn right, and begin walking back to the starting point, about four blocks away. This stretch of St. Claude includes even more cool places to stop, including ㉞ Fair Grinds Coffeehouse and ㉟ Carnaval Lounge, which hosts weekly comedy and burlesque shows, along with Latin music seven nights a week. The kitchen is run by Cozinha de Carnaval, which specializes in traditional Brazilian street food.

Although mostly a private event space, ㊱ The Art Garage, housed in an old auto body shop, hosts performances, live graffiti, and art exhibitions on the third Saturday night of every month. Just across Marigny Street from the Art Garage is the ㊲ Hi-Ho Lounge, where you can catch any number of local and national musical acts, from indie rock and hip-hop to funk and jazz. Another spot to consider as you make your way back to the starting point is ㊳ Kebab, which boasts an array of Middle Eastern dishes. Continue one and a half blocks back to St. Roch Market.

*The culinary and beverage options on St. Claude include the AllWays Lounge and Cabaret (left) and Nola Mia.*

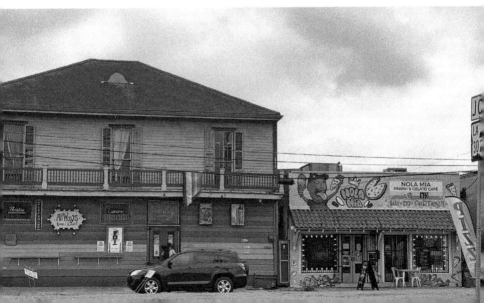

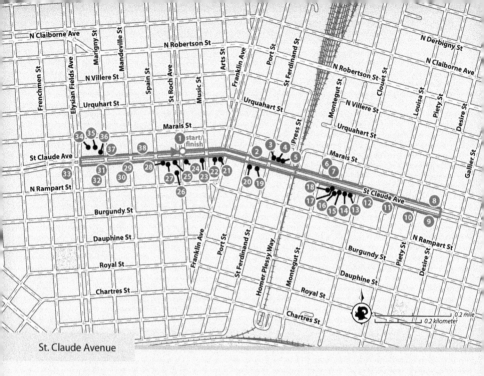

St. Claude Avenue

## Points of Interest

1. St. Roch Market  strochmarket.com, 2381 St. Claude Ave., 504-267-0388

2. Maypop Community Herb Shop  maypopherbshop.com, 2701 St. Claude Ave., 504-304-5067

3. Gerken's Bike Shop  gerkensbikeshop.com, 2803 St. Claude Ave., 504-373-6924

4. Poke-Chan  poke-chan.com, 2809 St. Claude Ave., 504-571-5446

5. Faubourg Wines  faubourgwines.com, 2805 St. Claude Ave., 504-342-2217

6. N7  n7nola.com, 1117 Montegut St.

7. Junction Bar & Grill  junctionnola.com, 3021 St. Claude Ave., 504-272-0205

8. Stuph'D Beignets and Burgers  5363 Franklin Ave., 504-459-4571

9. Rosalita's Backyard Tacos  3304 St. Claude Ave., 504-354-2468

10. Robert Emery Chocolate  robertemerychocolate.com, 1032 Piety St., 504-975-3239

11. Capt. Sal's Seafood and Chicken  captsalseafoodandchicken.com, 3168 St. Claude Ave., 504-948-9990

12. Art Space 3116  artspace3116.weebly.com, 3116 St. Claude Ave., 504-491-0598

(13) Galaxie  galaxietacos.com, 3060 St. Claude Ave., 504-827-1443

(14) Saint-Germain  saintgermainnola.com, 3054 St. Claude Ave., 504-218-8729

(15) Red's Chinese  redschinese.com, 3048 St. Claude Ave., 504-304-6030

(16) The Domino  dominola.com, 3044 St. Claude Ave., 504-354-8737

(17) The Grand Maltese  3040 St. Claude Ave., 504-330-1051

(18) The Get Down NOLA  the-get-down-nola.business.site, 3036 St. Claude Ave., 225-434-8500

(19) St. Coffee  facebook.com/stcoffeestclaude, 2718 St. Claude Ave.

(20) The New Movement  neworleanscomedy.wordpress.com, 2706 St. Claude Ave., 504-302-8264

(21) Chakras NOLA  facebook.com/chakrasnola, 1036 Franklin Ave., 504-266-2080

(22) Artisan Bar & Cafe  artisanbarneworleans.com, 2514 St. Claude Ave., 504-510-4340

(23) Morrow's  morrowsnola.com, 2438 St. Claude Ave., 504-827-1519

(24) Byrdie's Pottery  byrdiespottery.org, 2402A St. Claude Ave.

(25) New Orleans Healing Center  www.neworleanshealingcenter.org, 2372 St. Claude Ave., 504-940-1130

(26) Café Istanbul  cafeistanbulnola.com, 2372 St. Claude Ave., 504-975-0286

(27) New Orleans Boulder Lounge  climbnobl.com, 2360 St. Claude Ave., 504-962-7609

(28) Vintage Voyage  2348 St. Claude Ave., 214-876-5779

(29) Bao and Noodle  baoandnoodle.com, 2266 St. Claude Ave., 504-272-0004

(30) Arabella Casa di Pasta  arabellanola.com, 2258 St. Claude Ave., 504-533-9223

(31) AllWays Lounge and Cabaret  theallwayslounge.net, 2240 St. Claude Ave., 504-321-5606

(32) Nola Mia  nolamiallc.com, 2230 St. Claude Ave., 504-249-5009

(33) Baldwin & Co.  baldwinandcobooks.com, 1030 Elysian Fields Ave., 504-708-4804

(34) Fair Grinds Coffeehouse  fairgrinds.com, 2221 St. Claude Ave.

(35) Carnaval Lounge  carnavallounge.com, 2227 St. Claude Ave., 504-265-8855

(36) The Art Garage  artgarage.events, 2231 St. Claude Ave., 504-717-0750

(37) Hi-Ho Lounge  facebook.com/hi.ho.NOLA, 2239 St. Claude Ave., 504-945-4446

(38) Kebab  kebabnola.com, 2315 St. Claude Ave., 504-383-4328

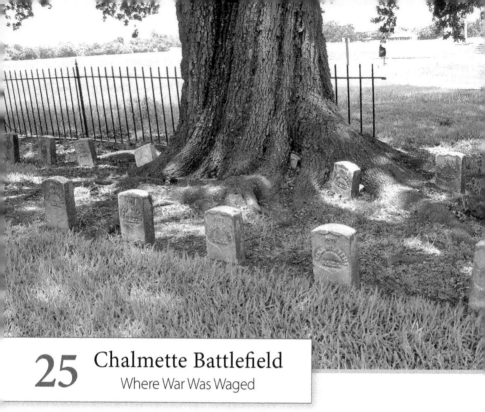

## 25 Chalmette Battlefield
### Where War Was Waged

*Above: Take some time to stroll through Chalmette National Cemetery, where more than 15,000 war veterans are buried.*

BOUNDARIES: St. Bernard Hwy., Mississippi River, Military Cemetery Rd., Battlefield Rd.
DISTANCE: 2 miles
PARKING: At the visitor center
PUBLIC TRANSIT: None, but the paddle wheeler *Creole Queen* travels here from the French Quarter.
  Visit creolequeen.com for more information.

As you drive down St. Bernard Highway, an industrial stretch of road dotted with oil refineries and chemical companies, it seems almost inconceivable that a decisive battle in the War of 1812 was fought just behind the Norfolk-Southern Railroad tracks in St. Bernard Parish, about 7 miles from downtown New Orleans.

The day was January 8, 1815, and Maj. Gen. Andrew Jackson's stunning victory over experienced British troops—in less than 2 hours—was considered the greatest American land victory of the War of 1812. The Battle of New Orleans not only preserved America's claim to the Louisiana Territory, it led to migration and settlement along the Mississippi River and made Jackson, who would go on to become the seventh president of the United States, a national hero.

One of six sites in Jean Lafitte National Historical Park and Preserve, Chalmette Battlefield tells the story of the war through exhibits and films at the visitor center, along with a 1.5-mile walk around the grounds and various other outdoor exhibits. Every January, the park brings the past to life with a living-history celebration featuring cannon and musket firings, period crafts and cooking, War of 1812 military drills and tactics, war reenactments, and an evening lantern tour. In January 2015, the battlefield celebrated its bicentennial with four days of activities.

Like other historical sites in and around New Orleans, this one is reputed to harbor spirits: many paranormal experts consider Chalmette one of the most haunted battlefields in the United States.

A few tips: Steer clear of small mounds of dirt, where fire ants may live. Don't climb the oak trees in the picnic area. Don't bring metal detectors on park property—relic hunting is strictly forbidden. And as you're walking, be on the lookout for cars, because this walk covers the same ground as the park's self-guided driving tour.

## Walk Description

Begin at the visitor center, where you can learn about the importance of the Battle of New Orleans in the War of 1812 through displays, maps, interactive exhibits, and films. The center's museum store sells books, period music, reproductions of war memorabilia, and children's books. Chalmette Battlefield sustained major damage in Hurricane Katrina; the visitor center was destroyed, and most of the structures were damaged. Although the battlefield reopened a year after the storm—in September 2006—it didn't fully recover until 2010, when the new visitor center was completed.

After exiting the visitor center, head a few feet to the left to Battlefield Tour Loop Road, a 1.5-mile roadway with stations where you can sit on a bench and read plaques that explain the war's major milestones. As you begin walking, look to your right at the Malus-Beauregard House, a restored Greek Revival mansion built nearly 20 years after the Battle of New Orleans. The house is named after its first and last owners—Madeleine Pannetier Malus in the 1830s and Judge René Beauregard (son of Confederate general P. G. T. Beauregard) in 1880. The National Park Service, which runs Chalmette Battlefield, bought the house in 1949.

Continue walking around the loop where you'll pass exhibits that explain the British battle plan, which called for attacks along the river, against the American rampart near the swamp, and on the west bank. Other exhibits explain the British artillery batteries, the roads and ditches used for the assault, and the march of the 93rd Highlanders across the battlefield. (The American line of defense is explained on the walkway leading into the park.)

At around the halfway point, you'll see a pathway leading to Chalmette National Cemetery. It's not included in this walk, but feel free to explore the grounds where more than 15,000 war veterans are buried. The cemetery was established in May 1864 as a final resting place for Union soldiers who died in Louisiana during the Civil War. The cemetery also includes the gravesites of veterans of the Spanish-American War, World Wars I and II, and the Vietnam War. Four Americans who fought in the War of 1812 are also buried in the cemetery, though only one of them took part in the Battle of New Orleans.

From the cemetery, continue circling around the loop to the area that served as the main attack of the British under Maj. Gen. Edward M. Pakenham, commander of the British army at Chalmette, and Maj. Gen. Samuel Gibbs. On January 8, 1815, Pakenham sent 7,000 troops head-on against the American position, concentrating their attack on the rampart's ends. But the American troops responded with devastating effect. Pakenham, Gibbs, and other high-ranking officers were killed or wounded, and the British soon surrendered.

Turn left on Battlefield Road, heading southwest. The story of the American line of defense is told in exhibits that run along the rampart and Rodriguez Canal. The exhibits describe American troops, their weapons, the 1815 landscape, and the last major battle of the War of 1812.

Circle past the west side of the Chalmette Monument, then head straight past the visitor center and take the path to the left. You'll come to a three-way intersection—take the path that forks right to the Spotts Monument, erected in honor of Maj. Samuel Spotts, who fired the first gun in the Battle of New Orleans. Between the Malus-Beauregard House (to your left) and the river (straight ahead), you'll see exhibits telling the stories of the land and the people who lived here after the battle, including the development of a thriving free African American community.

At the end of the walkway, turn around and follow it back to the three-way intersection; then make a quick right, followed by a quick left, to reach the Chalmette Monument. Walk around the 100-foot-tall obelisk, which pays homage to the troops of the Battle of New Orleans. The cornerstone honoring the American victory at New Orleans was laid in January 1840, within days after Andrew Jackson visited the field on the battle's 25th anniversary. The state of Louisiana began building the monument in 1855, and it was completed in 1908. If you're up to it, consider climbing its 122 interior steps to the viewing platform at the top. If you do, take your time—while the climb isn't overly strenuous, the steps and handrails may be slick in wet or humid weather. Children should be accompanied by an adult.

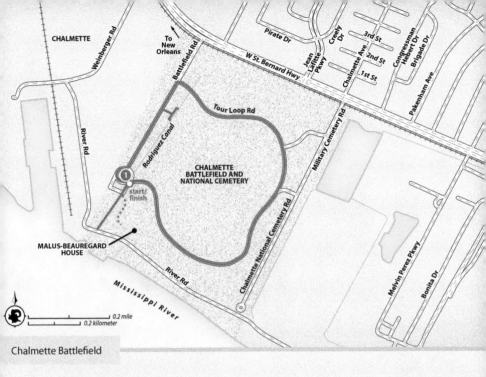

CHALMETTE

To New Orleans

Pirate Dr

Creely Dr

3rd St

Congressman Hebert Dr

Brigade Dr

Weinberger Rd

Battlefield Rd

W St. Bernard Hwy

Jean Lafitte Pkwy

Chalmette Ave

2nd St

1st St

Pakenham Ave

Tour Loop Rd

River Rd

Rodriguez Canal

CHALMETTE BATTLEFIELD AND NATIONAL CEMETERY

Military Cemetery Rd

start/ finish

Chalmette National Cemetery Rd

Melvin Perez Pkwy

Bonita Dr

MALUS-BEAUREGARD HOUSE

River Rd

Mississippi River

0.2 mile
0.2 kilometer

Chalmette Battlefield

## Point of Interest

1   Chalmette Battlefield and National Cemetery  nps.gov/jela/chalmette-battlefield.htm,
    8606 W. St. Bernard Hwy., Chalmette, 504-281-0510

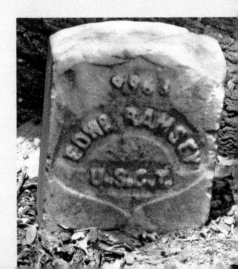

*Some of the tombstones in Chalmette National Cemetery date back to the mid-19th century.*

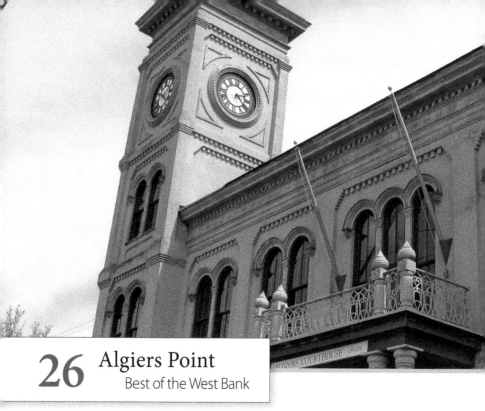

# 26 Algiers Point
### Best of the West Bank

*Above: The Algiers Courthouse was built in 1896 after the previous structure burned in the Great Fire of 1895.*

BOUNDARIES: Morgan St./Patterson Dr., Belleville St., Eliza St.
DISTANCE: 1.5 miles
PARKING: Free on the street, but check signs for time limits.
PUBLIC TRANSIT: Algiers–Canal Street ferry

Algiers Point is one of those "best kept secret" kinds of neighborhoods—one that mixes the charm and character of Uptown New Orleans with the affordability and quaintness of small-town America. For some house hunters, its location on the West Bank of the Mississippi River is an immediate turnoff. For others, it's the perfect landing spot.

Typically referred to as "the Point," Algiers Point is nestled within Algiers, the only part of New Orleans located on the West Bank. Listed on the National Register of Historic Places, it is the second-oldest neighborhood in New Orleans—the French Quarter is first—and while most of it was destroyed in the Great Fire of 1895, its rebuilt residences, from Creole cottages to Greek Revivals, give it the feel of a 19th-century village.

One of Algiers Point's biggest draws is the Algiers–Canal Street ferry, which runs all day long and can carry pedestrians and bicyclists to either side of the river in a matter of minutes. Residents often boast that they can get to downtown New Orleans more quickly than many who live on the East Bank.

The Point is also home to a number of bed-and-breakfasts, along with locally owned restaurants, music clubs, and cafés. Over the past few years, music festivals, art and farmers' markets, home tours, and other events have attracted locals and visitors alike.

## Walk Description

Begin at the Algiers–Canal Street ferry landing. If you've taken the ferry from downtown New Orleans, you've already noticed the spectacular view of the city's skyline. If you've traveled by car, walk to the top of the levee and take in its beauty. Also at the top of the levee is the ❶ Jazz Walk of Fame, a project of the New Orleans Jazz National Historic Park. The paved walkway features tributes to such jazz greats as Louis Armstrong, Jelly Roll Martin, and Al Hirt. Jazz plays an important role in the history of Algiers Point, with countless musicians having made their homes in this West Bank community. A free audio tour is available by calling 504-613-4062.

Take the stairs or ramp down to ground level. The ❷ Dry Dock Café, to the right, is an Algiers Point institution that offers a great selection of local brews, po'boys, and burgers. Next to the Dry Dock is ❸ Tavolino Pizza & Lounge, where pizzas range from a gorgonzola and date pizza to a pie topped with brie and prosciutto.

Turn left on Morgan Street, which turns into Patterson Drive (also known as the River Road). Check out the ❹ Algiers Courthouse, a Romanesque-style structure built in 1896 after the previous courthouse burned in the 1895 blaze. The courthouse houses a small-claims court, voter-registration and marriage-license offices, and other services. Behind the courthouse is a carriage house that was once home to a stable and jail. The Friends of the Algiers Courthouse assists the city of New Orleans in preserving and maintaining the property. Every spring, the group holds a crawfish-boil fundraiser to help in its preservation efforts.

Two doors from the courthouse, at 237 Morgan St., is the former home of jazz musician Emmett Hardy, a cornetist who died in 1925. Hardy played in Brownlee's Orchestra; the New Orleans Rhythm Kings; and with violinist Oscar Marcour, the Boswell Sisters, and drummer Arthur "Monk" Hazel. Hardy lived in the house from 1920 to 1923.

Continue walking down Morgan Street. The tall red building to the left is a luxury-condo development, one of the few modern structures to be built on the Point. Across the street, ⑤ **Beatrixbell Handcrafted Jewelry & Gift** sells an array of handcrafted jewelry and other hand-made wares.

Walk three blocks to the corner of Patterson Drive and Olivier Street. The ⑥ **Old Point Bar** is a haven for music lovers, with live performances almost every night. The bar features outdoor seating, pool tables and dart boards, and local brews. Across the street is Warren's Corner, a one-time Cajun restaurant now used as a special-events venue and an occasional film set.

At the Old Point Bar, turn right on Olivier Street and walk two blocks to Pelican Avenue, past beautifully landscaped and brightly painted homes, many designed in the Greek Revival style. At the corner of Olivier and Pelican is ⑦ **Mount Olivet Episcopal Church**. Founded in 1845, it is built entirely of cypress and, according to the church, has withstood several fires and hurricanes.

Turn left on Pelican Avenue and walk two blocks to Belleville Street. On the right, the ⑧ **Cita Dennis Hubbell Library** is New Orleans's oldest public library, having been built in 1907 with a donation from Andrew Carnegie. The library has seen its share of hard times, most notably in the 1960s when roof leaks, falling plaster, and buckling floors forced it to close. Because the city was building a new, more modern library in another part of Algiers about 4 miles away, officials decided to shut down the Algiers Point branch, much to the disappointment of neighborhood residents. It reopened in 1975 following a grassroots campaign led by resident and activist Cita Dennis Hubbell, who cited the building's architecture, history, and neighborhood convenience as reasons to save it. Hubbell had such an impact on the library's survival that it was renamed in her memory after she died in 2002.

Although the building escaped serious damage after Hurricane Katrina—it reopened after a couple of months—structural problems predating the storm shut it down again in 2008. The library operated out of a temporary branch at the Carriage House behind the Algiers Court-house, where it remained until July 2013, when a repaired Hubbell Library reopened for the third time.

Across Belleville Street from the library you'll see Belleville Assisted Living, a retirement community built on the site of the old Belleville School, which dates back to 1895. Turn right on Belleville, walk one block to Alix Street, turn right, and walk one block to Vallette Street.

Turn left on Vallette Street past the ⑨ **Appetite Repair Shop**, a to-go joint located on the ground floor of a raised shotgun house. Described by the shop's chef Pete Vazquez as "weird and wonderful," the shop has an ever-changing menu that often includes such dishes as Thai roast pork and spicy lamb gyro. Walk one block to the ⑩ **Rosetree Blown Glass Studio and Gallery**, at the corner of Vallette and Eliza Streets. Housed in the old Algy Theater, which has maintained its Art Deco look, the studio creates exquisite works of art—from perfume bottles to vases—using traditional glassblowing techniques. The gallery offers a viewing window where visitors can watch the artists at work.

Turn right and walk two blocks on Eliza Street to Verret Street, past ⓫ Trinity Lutheran Church on your right. Dating back to the mid-1870s, the church was organized by a group of German families in Algiers. The congregation's first house of worship was dedicated in 1876, the current Gothic/Colonial Revival–style church in 1911.

Turn right on Verret Street and walk one block to Alix Street, passing ⓬ McDonogh Park—also known as the Bermuda Triangle because it's bounded by Bermuda, Verret, and Alix Streets—on your left. In April 2013, the park received a long-awaited makeover, with volunteers painting signs, building wooden benches, and installing a new baseball diamond. The green space is also home to the Algiers War Memorial.

*The view of the New Orleans skyline from the West Bank of the Mississippi River in Algiers Point*

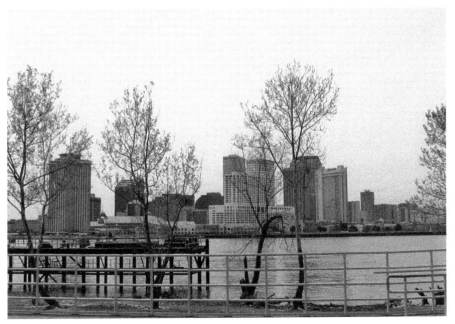

At the corner of Verret and Alix is **13** **Holy Name of Mary Church**, which was built in 1929 in the Tudor Gothic style. The church has more than 75 stained glass windows and marble and artwork from a previous church building.

Continue on Verret past the **14** **Tout de Suite Cafe**, an adorable eatery that's open for breakfast and lunch. At Verret Street and Pelican Avenue, **15** **Confetti Park** is a haven for the pint-size set. This pocket park has playground equipment and picnic tables under cypress trees, plus a fence with confetti-like cutouts. In 2000, residents joined together to form Confetti Kids, a nonprofit group that holds family-friendly events such as an Easter-egg hunt, a Spooktacular Halloween Party, and a Friendship Day Parade. The group's signature event is the Candy Land Ball and Fundraiser.

Continue on Verret to Delaronde Street and turn left. The house at 407 Delaronde is the one-time residence of jazz musician Norman Brownlee, a pianist and bandleader who died in 1967 and who lived at this address from 1912 to 1922. He was the leader of Brownlee's Orchestra, which also featured Emmett Hardy and Arthur "Monk" Hazel, among other musicians.

Walk one block to Lavergne Street and turn left; then walk one block to Pelican and turn right. A little more than a block ahead on your left, at 335 Pelican after you cross Bermuda Street, is **16** **House of the Rising Sun Bed and Breakfast**, which the owners named after the fictitious house of ill repute that the Animals made famous in their 1964 hit song. The house was built in 1896 after the original 1870 cottage burned down in the Great Fire of 1895.

Cross Seguin Street past **17** **Congregation Coffee**, a roastery and café. In this same block, on your right at 228 Pelican, is the one-time home of Mayor Martin Behrman, who served as New Orleans's leader for four consecutive terms from 1904 to 1920. He served again from 1925 to 1926, when he died in office at age 61. Today, there are streets, schools, and parks named after Behrman.

At the end of the block, on the corner of Pelican and Bouny Street, is the **18** **Crown & Anchor**, a British-style watering hole known for its Thursday-night pub quizzes, dart games, and an impressive selection of draft and bottled beers.

Turn right on Bouny and walk two blocks back to the ferry landing.

## Points of Interest

**1** Jazz Walk of Fame nps.gov/jazz, Algiers–Canal Street Ferry Terminal, 504-589-4841

**2** Dry Dock Café 133 Delaronde St., 504-361-8240

**3** Tavolino Pizza & Lounge facebook.com/TavolinoLounge, 141 Delaronde St., 504-605-3365

**4** Algiers Courthouse friendsofthealgierscourthouse.org, 225 Morgan St., 504-407-0435

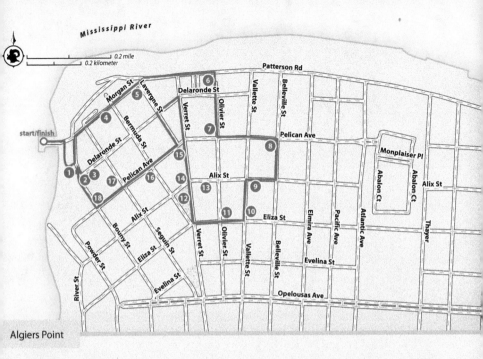

## Algiers Point

⑤ Beatrixbell Handcrafted Jewelry & Gift  beatrixbell.com/new-orleans-gift-shop, 337 Morgan St., 504-507-0955

⑥ Old Point Bar  oldpointbarnola.com, 545 Patterson Dr., 504-364-0950

⑦ Mount Olivet Episcopal Church  mountolivet.org, 530 Pelican Ave., 504-366-4650

⑧ Cita Dennis Hubbell Library  nolalibrary.org, 725 Pelican Ave., 504-596-3113

⑨ Appetite Repair Shop  appetiterepair.com, 400 Vallette St., 504-602-9990

⑩ Rosetree Blown Glass Studio  rosetreegallery.com, 446 Vallette St., 504-366-3602

⑪ Trinity Lutheran Church  620 Eliza St., 504-368-0411

⑫ McDonogh Park  Bounded by Bermuda, Verret, and Alix Streets

⑬ Holy Name of Mary Church  holynameofmarynola.org, 400 Verret St., 504-362-5511

⑭ Tout de Suite Cafe  toutdesuitecafe.com, 347 Verret St., 504-362-2264

⑮ Confetti Park  451 Pelican Ave. at Verret St.

⑯ House of the Rising Sun Bed and Breakfast  risingsunbnb.com, 335 Pelican Ave., 504-231-6498

⑰ Congregation Coffee  congregationcoffee.com, 240 Pelican Ave., 504-265-0194

⑱ Crown & Anchor English Pub  crownandanchorpub.com, 200 Pelican Ave., 504-227-1007

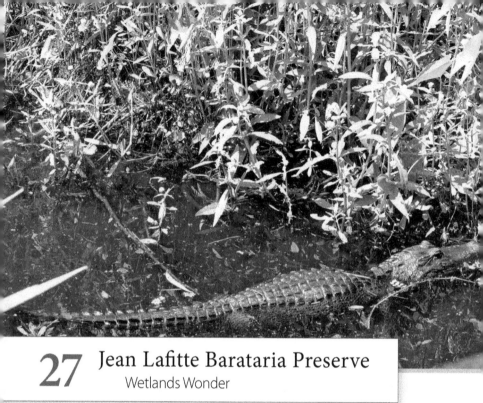

## 27   Jean Lafitte Barataria Preserve
### Wetlands Wonder

*Above: Alligators abound in the swamps of Jean Lafitte Barataria Preserve.*
*photo by Donna Goldenberg*

BOUNDARIES: Not applicable—this is an out-and-back walk on two trails within the preserve.
DISTANCE: 1.8 miles
PARKING: Free parking at trailhead
PUBLIC TRANSIT: None

You won't find swings, golf courses, or amusement park rides at Jean Lafitte National Historical Park's Barataria Preserve, but what you will find is one of the most stunning displays of nature that Louisiana has to offer.

With 23,000 acres of swamp, marsh, trails, and waterways, ❶ Barataria Preserve is a park like no other. On the West Bank of Jefferson Parish, about 20 miles from downtown New Orleans, it offers an up-close encounter with some of the state's endangered wetlands amid a setting of live oaks, bald cypress, palmettos, and wildflowers. Walk on any of the preserve's boardwalk or gravel trails, and you'll likely see a variety of wildlife from alligators and snakes to armadillos and nutria, not to mention more than 200 species of birds, among them pelicans and bald eagles.

That's not to say the park doesn't have its challenges. Hurricane Katrina destroyed or damaged 60% of the preserve's biggest trees, resulting in more light for invasive nonnative plants. The park's famous springtime iris blooms were especially affected, but the exquisite purple flowers are beginning to make a comeback.

The trails we've chosen are the Bayou Coquille Trail and the Marsh Overlook Trail, both of which are wheelchair-accessible and only about a mile from the visitor center. Be sure to stop at the center before you begin your hike. The center features dioramas, exhibits, a video, and a hands-on display. Park rangers are on hand to answer any questions you might have. In addition, the walk has seven stops, where you can phone 504-799-0802 to get an audio description of each one. (The following descriptions are based on the audio tour.)

Some tips to keep in mind before you begin: stay on boardwalks and trails, don't bring food or try to feed animals, don't pick flowers or dig up plants, and leave your pets at home. If you're taking the walk during the summer, bring a hat, insect repellent, and bottled water. And don't forget your camera and binoculars.

## Walk Description

Access the Bayou Coquille Trail from the Bayou Coquille parking lot, about a mile from the visitor center. The park recommends this trail to first-time visitors because it is one of the preserve's most diverse. It begins on high ground deposited by flooding from Bayou des Familles, once a major distributary of the Mississippi River. Dating back 2,000 years, it was once an American Indian village. The trail will take you through hardwood forest with live oaks, dwarf palmettos, bald cypress, and the freshwater marsh's floating prairie of grasses and aquatic plants.

Walk to Stop 1, where you'll be facing Bayou Coquille. *Coquille* is French for "shell," and the bayou got its name from the mounds of clamshells found here by early French surveyors. The discarded shells are evidence of a prehistoric Indian settlement, where Native Americans would consume small clams to supplement their diets of game, fish, and plants.

Walk to Stop 2 and take note of the live oaks. Live oaks are the densest, strongest wood native to North America. In the late 1700s and early 1800s, oak lumber was used to build warships. Live oaks typically grow thick trunks and wide-spreading limbs, and their low centers of gravity and extensive root systems help them resist high winds and storms. The trees at Barataria

Preserve are 250–400 years old and are reasonably healthy, though many have lost limbs in hurricanes or have been struck by lightning. Notice the resurrection ferns on the tree branches. In dry weather, they curl and turn brown. When it rains, the leaves unfurl and turn green.

Walk to Stop 3, where you'll learn the story of lumbering in Barataria from the 1880s to the 1920s. Loggers were especially attracted to bald cypress like the one in front of you. Bald cypress, which can grow up to 100 feet high and 15 feet in diameter, are resistant to rot and extremely durable. The logging process was grueling: loggers would cut the huge trees by hand with cross-cut saws, all while standing in mud and water and dealing with the threat of insects and snakes. Cables were then attached to the logs and dragged to the end of the canal, where they were bound together to make rafts, which then floated to the sawmill.

Walk to Stop 4, where you'll see a variety of invasive species of plants in the water below you, such as alligator weed, water hyacinth, and floating ferns called salvinia. They're called invasive because they are not native to Louisiana, having been brought by travelers from South America and Asia who did not realize the new plants would be destructive to the local environment. The invasive species have taken the place of native species such as wild iris and duckweed. Nutria, large rodents that call the preserve home, are also invasive species. They were brought to Louisiana in the 1930s for fur farming, replacing the native muskrats. The National Park Service has a program that aims to limit the growth of nonnative plant and animal species, but park rangers say it's impossible to eliminate them completely.

Walk to Stop 5, where you'll learn the important story of Louisiana's wetlands. Look across the canal to open marsh. Park officials say that if you return here in a few years, some of the marshland may be gone. Surges from tropical storms and hurricanes destroy vegetation, and rebuilding land or at least slowing the rate of the land's disappearance is a massive project.

Walk to Stop 6. One of the thrills of the Barataria Preserve trails is spotting alligators in the swamps. There's a healthy population of gators here, though some may be harder to spot than others. Although they can grow to up to 16 feet long, the longest alligators here are about 13 feet long. Alligators, along with the swamp's other animals and plants, are protected by law.

At the half-mile point, you'll enter the Marsh Overlook Trail, which is situated atop a bank that was formed by dredged material from the Kenta Canal. Once used for irrigating and draining plantation fields, the canal was deepened and widened in the late 19th century so loggers could gain access to the bald-cypress swamp.

Walk to Stop 7, where you'll learn that the grassland in the distance is actually a freshwater marsh that is not connected to the soil but is rather a floating mat of plants called a flotant. The marsh rises and falls with the water beneath it and is especially affected by wind direction and

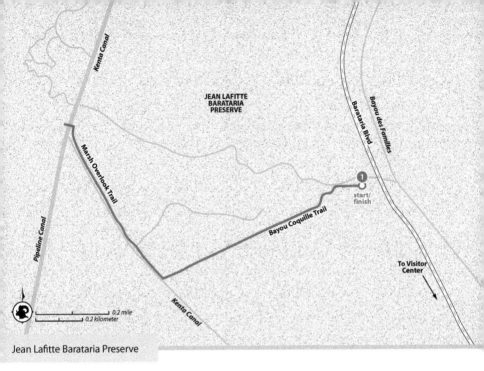

Jean Lafitte Barataria Preserve

rainfall. Among the wildlife that call the flotant home are rabbits, alligators, raccoons, nutria, coyotes, white-tailed deer, and many species of birds.

Turn around at the end of the Marsh Outlook Trail and make your way back to the beginning of the Bayou Coquille Trail. If you're up to it, check out some of the park's other trails, or save them for your next visit.

## Point of Interest

1. Barataria Preserve, Jean Lafitte National Historical Park  nps.gov/jela/barataria-preserve.htm, 6588 Barataria Blvd., Marrero, 504-689-3690, Ext. 10

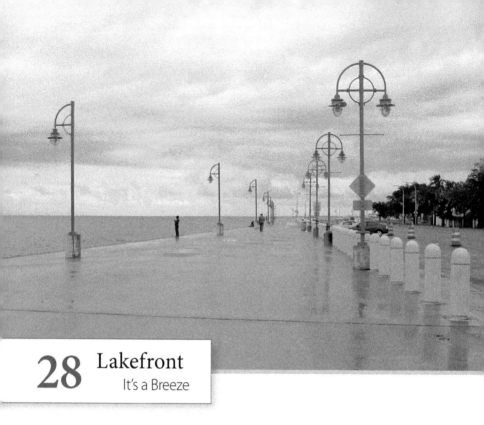

# 28 Lakefront
### It's a Breeze

*Above: Lakeshore Drive, which runs along Lake Pontchartrain, is the perfect place to take in a sunset and view passing boats.*

BOUNDARIES: Robert E. Lee Blvd., Lakeshore Dr., Marconi Dr.
DISTANCE: 3.1 miles
PARKING: Free parking on Robert E. Lee, in surrounding neighborhood, and at shopping-center parking lot
PUBLIC TRANSIT: RTA Bus #45 (Lakeview)

The Lakefront area may not hold the popularity of the Garden District or the French Quarter, but avid walkers consider it one of the most refreshing and invigorating places to take a stroll. That is especially true of Lakeshore Drive, which meanders several miles along Lake Pontchartrain, the Crescent City's most expansive body of water and a sort of home-away-from-home for local boating enthusiasts.

Lake Pontchartrain covers a 630-square-foot area, has an average depth of 14–16 feet, and touches six different parishes (counties). The lake is part of the Lake Pontchartrain Basin, which comprises numerous bodies of water that connect to the Gulf of Mexico through the Mississippi River.

Over the years, the lake has seen its share of environmental challenges, among them urban runoff, saltwater intrusion, and wetlands loss. In 1989, the nonprofit Lake Pontchartrain Basin Foundation, now the Pontchartrain Conservancy, was established to essentially save the lake. Its efforts have and continue to pay off. Seasonal swimming is allowed in designated areas, and water quality is monitored and publicized weekly at scienceforourcoast.org.

Every year, the conservancy sponsors a number of events, with proceeds going toward its various preservation and educational programs, including a day at the New Canal Lighthouse Museum, where children can engage in climate science and water quality activities. Every September, volunteer groups come together for the annual Beach Sweep, a massive cleanup effort.

## Walk Description

Start at the intersection of Lakeshore Drive and Robert E. Lee Boulevard. Stay on the east side of Lakeshore and head north toward the lake. About a block down is Lake Marina Drive, where the Orleans Marina is located. Lake Marina Drive leads to West End Park, a 30-acre green space around which sits the Southern Yacht Club and the New Orleans Municipal Yacht Harbor. For years, West End Park was home to a bustling seafood restaurant industry, but a series of storms and hurricanes over the years—including Katrina—wiped it out.

Continue walking along Lakeshore Drive past several restaurants to your left. ❶ Felix's Restaurant and Oyster Bar boasts oysters harvested from Louisiana's best oyster beds. ❷ The Blue Crab opened in 2013 as a dream by its owners to bring waterfront dining back to the neighborhood. ❸ Landry's has been around longer, and its views of Lake Pontchartrain are simply breathtaking.

As Lakeshore bends to the right, you'll see Louisiana's only working lighthouse. In 2005, the lighthouse was severely damaged in Hurricanes Katrina and Rita, but the Pontchartrain Conservancy has since rebuilt and transformed it into the ❹ New Canal Lighthouse Museum and Education Center. The center offers programs on the history of the lighthouse, the ecology of the Pontchartrain Basin, and the critical coastal issues facing South Louisiana.

Continue walking along Lakeshore Drive. To the right is the lakefront park, which, with its playgrounds, picnic shelters, and picnic pavilions, is the ideal place to spend a lazy weekend afternoon. Feel free to cross Lakeshore and get a closer view of the lake. But be extra-cautious because this is a busy street.

One of the highlights of the walk—besides the lake itself—is the famed Mardi Gras Fountain, between Canal Boulevard and Marconi Drive. Like the Lighthouse, the fountain sustained severe damage in Katrina but is now back to its original splendor. First built in 1960, the fountain is surrounded by plaques depicting the crests of Carnival organizations and krewes, including Rex, Bacchus, and Endymion.

Continue walking on Lakeshore, cross the Orleans Avenue Canal, and turn right on Marconi Drive. Walk down the steps on the left side of the street. You are now in the Lake Vista subdivision, which, along with West and East Lakeshore and Lake Terrace, makes up the lakefront's residential area. Lake Vista is the most interesting of the three areas, its design based on the Garden City movement under which all interior streets end in culs-de-sac and separate pedestrian lanes meet at the center of the development.

Walk eight blocks to Robert E. Lee Boulevard. Notice that the streets of Lake Vista are named for birds, such as Hawk and Swan, and the lanes for flowers, such as Azalea and Daisy. The neighborhood sustained substantial damage in Katrina, and many homes were rebuilt higher and sturdier.

At Robert E. Lee, turn right and continue walking over the Orleans Avenue Canal toward Canal Boulevard. Cross Canal and walk back to your starting point, just past ⑤ Mount Carmel Academy, one of the city's oldest and most respected Catholic high schools. At the strip shopping center to your right on Robert E. Lee, you have a few options for refreshments: ⑥ Chateau Café; ⑦ PJ's Coffee, inside Robért Fresh Market; and ⑧ Smoothie King. Across the street, you'll find ⑨ Celtica French Bakery, where the menu includes quiches, croissants, cream puffs, and eclairs.

*The historic New Canal Lighthouse on Lake Pontchartrain was established in 1839.*

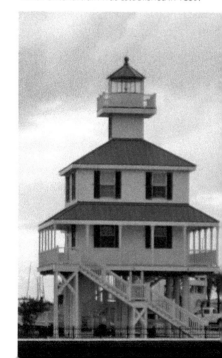

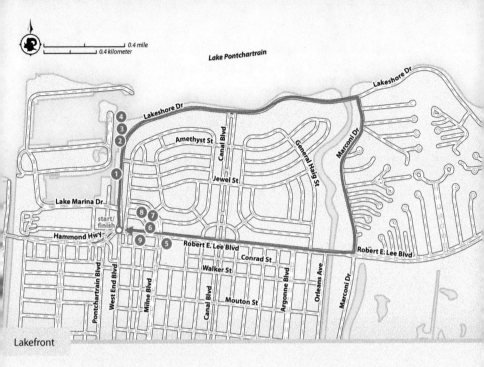

Lakefront

## Points of Interest

① Felix's Restaurant and Oyster Bar  felixs.com, 7400 Lakeshore Dr., 504-304-4125

② The Blue Crab  thebluecrabnola.com, 7900 Lakeshore Dr., 504-284-2898

③ Landry's Seafood  landrysseafood.com, 8000 Lakeshore Dr., 504-283-1010

④ New Canal Lighthouse Museum and Education Center  scienceforourcoast.org,
8001 Lakeshore Dr., 504-282-2134

⑤ Mount Carmel Academy  mcacubs.com, 7027 Milne St., 504-288-7626

⑥ Chateau Café  chateaucafenola.com, 139 Robert E. Lee Blvd., 504-286-1777

⑦ PJ's Coffee at Robért Fresh Market  pjscoffee.com, 153 Robert E. Lee Blvd., 504-282-3428

⑧ Smoothie King  smoothieking.com, 111 Robert E. Lee Blvd., 504-286-1471

⑨ Celtica French Bakery  facebook.com/celticafrenchbakery, 218 Robert E. Lee Blvd.

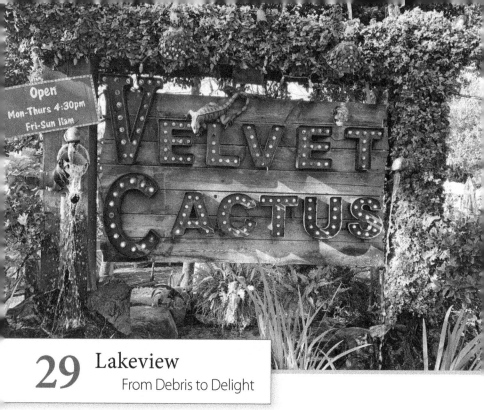

## 29 Lakeview
### From Debris to Delight

*Above: Velvet Cactus boasts one of the nicest outdoor dining spaces in New Orleans.*

BOUNDARIES: West End Blvd., Filmore Ave. Canal Blvd., Harrison Ave.
DISTANCE: 2.51 miles
PARKING: Free on the street and the Harrison Ave. neutral ground
PUBLIC TRANSIT: RTA Bus #45 (Lakeview)

Imagine your neighborhood wiped out by a powerful hurricane, its winds ripping off roofs and water from a nearby levee breach reaching as high as 9 feet.

Residents of Lakeview didn't have to imagine it—they lived it. On August 29, 2005, Hurricane Katrina obliterated this upper-middle-class community, destroying its homes along with its quality of life. Many residents drowned, unable or unwilling to evacuate in the days leading up to the storm.

While many survivors relocated to other parts of the country or to less-affected parts of New Orleans, others vowed to rebuild. Improvements in levee strength and flood control helped their cause, and today the neighborhood is as strong and vibrant as ever.

Lakeview is considered one of the most family-friendly areas of New Orleans, and most residents have no qualms about taking an evening stroll to Harrison Avenue, where they can shop at Lakeview Grocery, grab dinner at Velvet Cactus, or splurge on an ice-cream cone at the Creole Creamery.

Activities abound in Lakeview as well, from church and school fairs to the monthly Harrison Avenue Marketplace, sponsored by the Friends of Lakeview and the Lakeview Civic Improvement Association. The event features an art market, music, and food from area restaurants.

## Walk Description

Begin this walk at ❶ New Basin Canal Park at the intersection of West End Boulevard and Harrison Avenue. The linear park stretches 1.5 miles from Veterans Boulevard to Robert E. Lee Boulevard between West End and Pontchartrain Boulevards. The park features biking and walking trails, old-style lampposts, and benches. The park sits on what was once a shipping canal that operated from the 1830s to the 1940s from Lake Pontchartrain through swampland to what is now the Central Business District of New Orleans.

Walk six blocks to Filmore Avenue, turn right, and walk seven blocks to Canal Boulevard. As you walk, imagine the piles of debris that littered the neighborhood during the Katrina recovery process. Many residents lived in trailers provided by the Federal Emergency Management Agency, and for a long time, Lakeview resembled a mammoth mobile-home park.

Turn right on Canal Boulevard, an extension of the famed Canal Street, which runs from City Park Avenue to the Mississippi River. Canal Boulevard is largely a residential thoroughfare divided by a parklike neutral ground (New Orleans's version of a median). Due to the breach of the 17th Street Canal—on the west side of Lakeview—no one escaped the Katrina flooding in this neighborhood. Consequently, houses were either restored or built anew. It's easy to spot the newer ones: many are two- and three-story mansions, some of which dwarf their neighbors. Others are restored early-20th-century cottages and bungalows. Almost all of the houses were built high off the ground.

Walk four blocks to the intersection of Canal and Harrison Avenue, just past ❷ Lakeview Pearl, a sushi bar and Asian bistro. Cross Canal and continue walking along Harrison Avenue, the main commercial corridor of Lakeview. First up on Harrison is the ❸ Robert E. Smith Library, one of 14 branches of the New Orleans Public Library. Like the rest of Lakeview, the old library was flooded so badly that it had to be rebuilt from the ground up. The process took more than six years, but when the new building finally opened, it was bigger and better than ever. In addition to 40,000 volumes, the 12,700-square-foot library has a colorful, fully stocked children's corner, 17 computers, meeting space, and a self-checkout system.

Continuing on Harrison, walk two blocks to Memphis Street. To the left is ❹ St. Dominic Catholic Church, one of the largest in New Orleans. St. Dominic's parish dates back to 1924, though Lakeview's first formal place of Catholic worship—a small wooden chapel on nearby Chapelle Street—opened in 1912. As Lakeview grew, so did St. Dominic's need for a larger worship space, and in 1961 it moved to its current location on Harrison. Behind it is St. Dominic Catholic School, which serves students in prekindergarten through grade seven. One of the most memorable days in the church's history occurred on November 27, 2005, when St. Dominic held its first Mass three months after Katrina. The church had been gutted, and there was still no electricity or residents in Lakeview. But that didn't matter to church parishioners, who came from far and wide to attend the service. "This is the nucleus that holds this community together, and this is the nucleus that's going to bring the community back," a parishioner told USA Today.

Over the next several blocks you'll pass several commercial establishments, including ❺ Junior's on Harrison, a self-described neighborhood joint, which, in addition to burgers and fries, serves such fare as lemongrass brussels sprouts, honey citrus tacos, and Thai peanut salad. ❻ Gail's Fine Ice Cream is just behind it on Memphis Street.

Cross Memphis Street and continue past ❼ Lakeview Grocery, which has its own café, Harrison Cove, and regularly holds barbecues, seafood boils, and fish fries. On Sundays, the market hosts a waffle bar brunch. Other restaurants on this side of Harrison include ❽ Tastee, ❾ Three B's, and ❿ The Velvet Cactus, a Mexican eatery, which has an expansive outdoor patio perfect for sipping a pineapple-cilantro margarita or any number of other tropical drinks. Inside, the walls are adorned with the works of local artists, and most of the art is for sale.

Cross Harrison at Argonne Boulevard and turn right onto the other side of Harrison. As you cross, take note of the building to your left: that's ⓫ Edward Hynes Charter School, long one of the city's top-rated public schools. After Katrina, the original school building was torn down to make way for a new state-of-the-art campus. Students, at least those who returned to New Orleans, were schooled in temporary quarters while construction ensued. When the new Hynes opened more than six years after the storm, it was considered a crucial step in the neighborhood's recovery.

As you continue along Harrison, you'll pass an assortment of businesses, from salons to banks. The neighborhood fire station is on Harrison, and tucked down some of the side streets are spas, sweet shops, and doctor's offices. Over the next several blocks, from Harrison back to

Canal Boulevard, you'll also find that there are no shortages of places to dine, snack, or drink. There's ⑫ Dixie Chicken & Ribs, on Argonne just off Harrison; ⑬ Nola Snow Snoballs; and ⑭ Elle J's, which specializes in classic Italian. In the next block you'll pass a strip of businesses that includes ⑮ The Steak Knife, a neighborhood steakhouse; ⑯ Reginelli's Pizzeria, part of a local pizza chain; ⑰ Lakeview Burgers and Seafood; and ⑱ Parlay's, a legendary corner bar that claims to have the longest bar in New Orleans, at 60 feet.

If it's sweets you're craving, check out ⑲ Nola Beans, ⑳ the Creole Creamery, or ㉑ Sweet Life Bakery. And be sure to drop by ㉒ Little Miss Muffin (766 Harrison), a whimsical boutique next door to Nola Beans that sells everything from children's clothing to home-decor items.

At the corner of Canal and Harrison is ㉓ St. Paul's Episcopal Church and School, which got its start in a small room at Lee Circle in downtown New Orleans in the 1830s. Like St. Dominic's, St. Paul's moved several times before settling into its current digs on Canal Boulevard. It struggled to survive after Katrina, as illustrated on its website: "For three weeks the church and school sat under eight feet of polluted water and debris. The result was the total destruction of the first-floor interiors as well as two single-story buildings that had to be demolished. With 80 percent of the city flooded and businesses ruined, the tragic scattering of our people ensued. "With the help of volunteers from around the country, St. Paul's plunged into the rebuilding process, transforming mountains of debris into a source of pride. But it didn't just help itself—it helped all of Lakeview, opening a Homecoming Center to help restore lives and rebuild homes. Today, its services include raising money for communities that have experienced similar disasters.

Cross Canal Boulevard and continue six blocks to the starting point. Although this part of Lakeview is largely residential, it has seen major commercial growth in recent years, most notably on Harrison. It includes restaurants such as ㉔ Another Broken Egg, ㉕ District Donuts, Sliders, Brew, ㉖ Francesca Deli, and ㉗ El Gato Negro, along with such shops as ㉘ Little Pnuts Toy Shoppe and ㉙ Swoon. At the corner of Harrison and West End Boulevard is ㉚ Chris's Specialty Foods, a Cajun butcher shop where, among other things, you can get Louisiana meat pies, alligator sausage, and turducken—a chicken stuffed in a duck stuffed in a turkey.

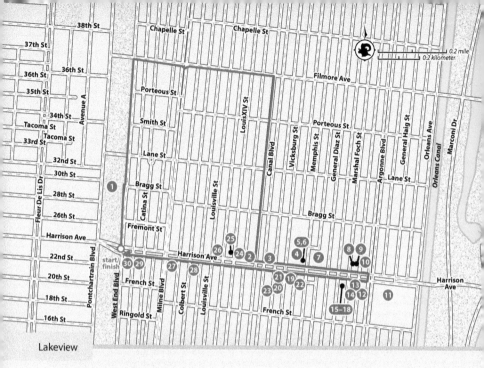

## Points of Interest

**1** New Basin Canal Park  Bounded by West End Blvd., Harrison Ave., Pontchartrain Blvd., and Filmore Ave.

**2** Lakeview Pearl  lakeviewpearl.com, 6300 Canal Blvd., 504-309-5711

**3** Robert E. Smith Library  nolalibrary.org, 6301 Canal Blvd., 504-596-2638

**4** St. Dominic Catholic Church  775 Harrison Ave., 504-482-4156

**5** Junior's on Harrison  juniorsonharrison.com, 789 Harrison Ave., 504-766-6902

**6** Gail's Fine Ice Cream  gailsfineicecream.com, 789 Harrison Ave., Suite B, 504-766-6902

**7** Lakeview Grocery  lakeviewgrocery.com, 801 Harrison Ave., 504-293-1201

**8** Tastee Restaurant  facebook.com/TasteeRestaurant, 901 Harrison Ave., 504-483-9080

**9** Three B's Burger and Wine Bar  threebs.com, 911 Harrison Ave., 504-249-8025

**10** The Velvet Cactus  thevelvetcactus.com, 6300 Argonne Blvd., 504-301-2083

**11** Edward Hynes Charter School  hynesschool.com, 990 Harrison Ave., 504-324-7160

**12** Dixie Chicken & Ribs  dixiechickenandribs.com, 6264 Argonne Blvd., 504-488-1377

**13** Nola Snow Snoballs  nolasnow.com, 908 Harrison Ave., 504-373-6555

(14) Elle J's  ellejslakeview.com, 900 Harrison Ave., 504-459-2262

(15) The Steak Knife  steakkniferestaurant.com, 888 Harrison Ave., 504-488-8981

(16) Reginelli's Pizzeria  reginellis.com, 874 Harrison Ave., 504-488-0133

(17) Lakeview Burgers and Seafood  lakeviewburgersandseafood.com, 872 Harrison Ave., 504-289-1032

(18) Parlay's Bar  facebook.com/parlays, 870 Harrison Ave., 504-304-6338

(19) Nola Beans  nolabeans.com, 762 Harrison Ave., 504-267-0783

(20) The Creole Creamery  creolecreamery.com, 6260 Vicksburg St., 504-482-2924

(21) The Sweet Life Bakery  nolasweetlife.com, 6268 Vicksburg St., 504-371-5153

(22) Little Miss Muffin  shoplittlemissmuffin.com, 766 Harrison Ave., 504-482-8200

(23) St. Paul's Episcopal Church and School  stpaulsnola.org, 6249 Canal Blvd., 504-488-3749

(24) Another Broken Egg Cafe  anotherbrokenegg.com, 607 Harrison Ave., 504-301-4667

(25) District Donuts, Sliders, Brew  districtdonuts.com, 527 Harrison Ave., 504-827-1152

(26) Francesca Deli  francescadeli.com, 515 Harrison Ave., 504-266-2511

(27) El Gato Negro  elgatonegronola.com  300 Harrison Ave., 504-488-0107

(28) Little Pnuts Toy Shoppe  littlepnuts.com, 400 Harrison Ave., 504-267-5083

(29) Swoon  swoonboutiquenola.com, 130 Harrison Ave., 504-516-2770

(30) Chris's Specialty Foods  chrisspecialtyfoods.com, 6251 West End Blvd., 504-309-0010

*New Basin Canal Park is a linear green space that runs between West End and Pontchartrain Boulevards in Lakeview.*

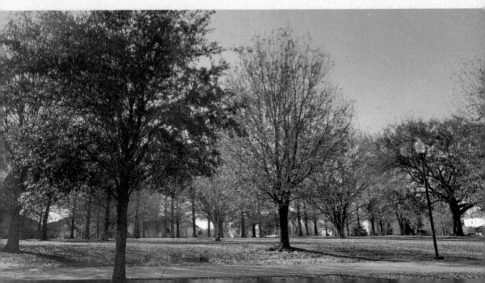

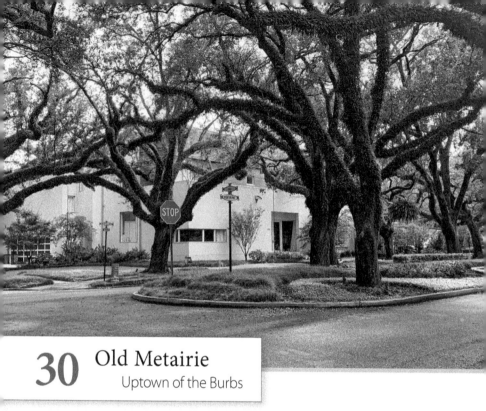

# 30 Old Metairie
## Uptown of the Burbs

BOUNDARIES: Friederichs Ave., Northline St., Woodvine Ave., Duplessis St., Metairie Road
DISTANCE: 1.91 miles
PARKING: Street parking
PUBLIC TRANSIT: Unavailable

Take a stroll down Northline Street in Old Metairie, and if you didn't know any better, you'd swear you were in one of the poshest parts of New Orleans. Think St. Charles Avenue, or the Garden District, where one mansion is more elegant than the next.

Old Metairie, developed in the 1920s, is part of unincorporated Metairie, which like the typical American suburb has more than its share of strip malls, chain restaurants, and big-box stores. For the most part, the neighborhoods are pleasant and welcoming, and as you get closer to Lake Pontchartrain, even palatial and grandiose.

But none are nearly as magnificent and breathtaking as the Metairie Club Gardens section of Old Metairie. Northline. Pelham. Nassau. Woodvine. Take a stroll down any of the streets that make up this neighborhood in Jefferson Parish, just west of New Orleans, and you'll be glad you ventured into the burbs.

# Walk Description

Begin the walk in front of Friederichs Square at the corner of Friederichs Avenue and Metairie Road, the area's main drag. ❶ Royal Blend Coffee & Tea is a popular neighborhood hangout. The strip includes several upscale shops, including ❷ Elizabeth's Clothing, ❸ Sorellas, and ❹ Dolce.

Turn right on Friederichs and walk three blocks to oak-canopied Northline, a stately drive flanked by million-dollar-plus mansions, both new and old. As stated earlier, Northline is one of the most picturesque and prestigious streets in the entire New Orleans metropolitan area, if not the state. Its stately homes include the ultramodern, Greek Revival, and English Tudor.

From Friederichs, walk five blocks to Woodvine Avenue. Just off Northline are Pelham Avenue and Nassau Drive, both of which rival Northline in terms of beauty and magnificence. Feel free to detour around those streets, which will bring you back to Northline.

At the intersection of Northline and Woodvine is ❺ Metairie Country Club, a private club that opened in 1922 as the neighborhood was beginning to take shape. Turn right and walk one block down Woodvine to just past Geranium St. Woodvine splits off to the left, but keep going straight along Park Road to Duplessis Street. Just ahead is ❻ Metairie Park Country Day School, one of the Crescent City's most exclusive private schools. Established in 1929, Country Day is a coeducational, independent school for students in prekindergarten through 12th grade. The school is known for its rigorous curriculum, use of advanced technology, and innovative approaches to learning.

Turn right on Duplessis and walk two blocks to Hector Avenue. Turn left on Hector and walk to Frisco Avenue, which runs alongside the infamous Old Metairie train tracks. The tracks are infamous because of how often—and how long—they back up traffic at crossings, especially at Metairie Road, a heavily used commuter roadway.

Turn right on Frisco and walk a block to Metairie Road, the neighborhood's commercial corridor. Metairie Road actually stretches just over 3 miles from the Pontchartrain Expressway to Severn Avenue. It is home to dozens of shops, restaurants, salons, cafés, and other businesses, and the neighborhoods on both sides of the road are worthy of a stroll. But it might be best known for the St. Patrick's Day Parade that wows throngs of green-laden revelers every year on the Sunday before March 17. Feel free to cross the tracks (after looking both ways) and explore the rest of Metairie Road on your own.

If you're in need of a break, consider a stop at ⑦ Winston's Pub & Patio, a neighborhood institution where you can grab a beer or cocktail along with an order of loaded fries or meat pies. Along Metairie Road you'll find a plethora of upscale boutiques such as ⑧ Cella's, ⑨ FeBe Too, ⑩ Nola Boo, ⑪ Bella Bella, and ⑫ Iron Horse Clothier.

Continue down Metairie Road past ⑬ St. Francis Xavier Catholic Church and School, part of the Archdiocese of New Orleans. Every year, the church holds an array of neighborhood events, such as Trunk or Treat, a holiday craft market, and a crawfish boil. Just past the church is ⑭ Jade, an interior and design store that sells a variety of kitchen, bath, and dining wares.

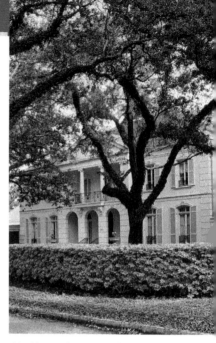

*Northline and its surrounding streets are lined with mansions such as this one near posh Vincent Avenue.*

As you return to the starting point two blocks away, you'll pass several more shops, including ⑮ Little Miss Muffin and ⑯ Em's. To the left, you'll also see one of the best public schools in Louisiana—⑰ Metairie Academy for Advanced Studies, an elementary magnet school for gifted children in grades pre-K–5.

## Points of Interest

① Royal Blend Coffee & Tea  royalblendcoffee.com, 204 Metairie Road, 504-835-7779

② Elizabeth's Clothing  204 Metairie Road, 504-833-3717

③ Sorellas  sorellasnola.com, 200 Metairie Road, 504-265-0011

④ Dolce  facebook.com/shopdolceboutique, 204 Metairie Road, 504-609-2222

⑤ Metairie Country Club  metairiecc.org, 580 Woodvine Ave., 504-833-4671

⑥ Metairie Park Country Day School  mpcds.com, 300 Park Road, 504-837-5204

⑦ Winston's Pub & Patio  winstonspubandpatio.com, 531 Metairie Road, 504-831-8705

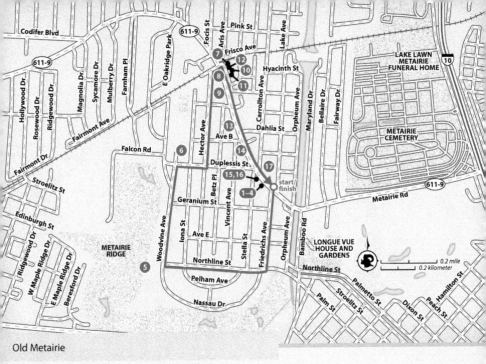

Old Metairie

8 Cella's Boutique  shopcellas.com, 512 Metairie Road, 504-407-3828

9 FeBe Too  febeclothing.com, 474 Metairie Road, 504-835-5250

10 Nola Boo  nolaboo.payscapecommerce.com, 517 Metairie Road, 504-510-4655

11 Bella Bella  bellabellashop.com  501 Metairie Road, 504-834-2009

12 Iron Horse Clothier  ironhorsenola.com, 523 Metairie Road, 504-644-4800

13 St. Francis Xavier Catholic Church and School  stfrancisxavier.com, 105 Vincent Ave., 504-835-6809

14 Jade  jadenola.com, 324 Metairie Road, 504-875-4420

15 Little Miss Muffin  shoplittlemissmuffin.com, 246 Metairie Road, 504-834-2795

16 Em's Boutique  246 Metairie Road, 504-834-2795

17 Metairie Academy for Advanced Studies  jpschools.org/metairie, 201 Metairie Road, 504-833-5539

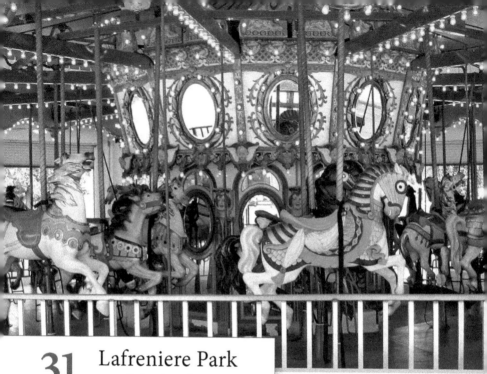

# 31 Lafreniere Park
## Suburban Sanctuary

*Above: The carousel at Lafreniere Park boasts 30 moving horses, a tiger, a zebra, and two chariots.*

BOUNDARIES: David Dr., Wytchwood Dr., Madewood Dr., Park Manor Dr., Judith St., W. Napoleon Ave.
DISTANCE: 1.5 miles
PARKING: Free parking throughout park
PUBLIC TRANSIT: Jefferson Transit Bus E1 (Veterans)

Big-box stores, chain restaurants, and strip shopping centers—they pretty much define Veterans Memorial Boulevard in Metairie, a sprawling suburb just west of New Orleans. But thanks to the efforts of a citizens' group back in the early 1970s, the 155-acre ❶ Lafreniere Park was born, becoming the center of recreational life in what would become one of the most populous areas of southern Louisiana. Named after Nicolas Chauvin de la Frénière, a former Louisiana attorney general who inherited the land in the mid-18th century, the park opened in 1982, after voters approved a bond issue to acquire the land.

Over the past three decades, the park has evolved into a destination, inviting tourists and locals alike to take in its fountains, lagoons, gardens, and trails. Among the park's highlights is a boardwalk through Marsh Island, a wildlife habitat where visitors can easily spot such species as ibis, sandpipers, geese, swans, and egret. For children, the park offers a 4,000-square-foot spray park and an old-fashioned carousel. If they play soccer, chances are they'll be competing at Lafreniere, which has five soccer fields and four softball fields. The park also features a gated dog park called Bark Park, a disc golf course, and a 2-mile jogging path.

Lafreniere is home to some of the area's most popular holiday events, including the Uncle Sam Jam, a Fourth of July extravaganza; Park-a-Boo, a Halloween shindig for children; and Holiday in the Park, a spectacular Christmas-light display with a 60-foot sea serpent in the lagoon, a princess and her magical castle, and the gingerbread man. Every year, the park also hosts Lafreniere Live, a concert series at the Al Copeland Meadow Concert Stage, named after the late founder of Popeye's, the fried chicken chain founded in New Orleans in 1972.

## Walk Description

From Veterans Memorial Boulevard, drive south on Downs Boulevard, cross over North Scenic Drive, and pull into the parking lot to the left. Start off by walking southwest along Downs across from the park's soccer fields. To the left is the first of many lakes that you'll see as you make your way around the park. Benches surround the lake, making it a pleasant spot to read a book or pose for photos.

Walk past the lake and turn left. Continue walking and cross the first bridge. This will take you to the concert pavilion, where many festivals take place. Turn south at the pavilion toward the lake, where ducks and other waterfowl make their home. Circle around until you see another bridge. This one leads to a circular garden, where markers tell the history of the park. This is also the location of the Compassionate Friends Memorial Garden. Each year, Compassionate Friends, a nonprofit support group for parents and families who have lost a child, holds a memorial walk in the park.

Continue walking south until you reach the park's boardwalk bridge, which winds through Marsh Island, a natural wildlife habitat. Listen for the sounds of crickets, ducks, and the occasional crowing rooster. Squirrels, turtles, rabbits, raccoons, nutria, and opossums also call the island home. In the middle of the boardwalk is a small pavilion where you can stop and marvel at the sight of geese, swans, and ducks floating in the lake.

As you step off the boardwalk, don't be surprised to encounter ducks, ibis, and other wildlife hanging out on the pathways and the shores of the lake. Continue circling until you see a trash receptor to the right. Turn right, walk a few feet to the jogging trail, and take another right on

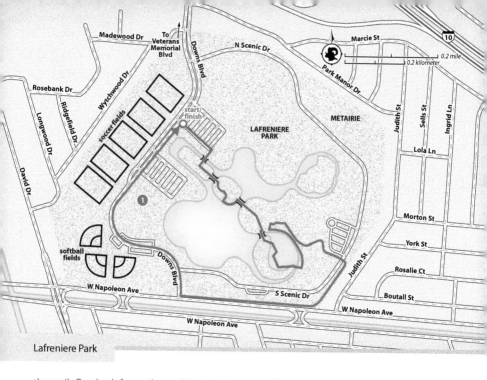

Lafreniere Park

the trail. On the left are the park's administrative offices and the Foundation Room, the park's special-events venue.

Cross South Scenic Drive and continue on the jogging trail. Be wary of joggers, who tend to pack the park on weekends. As you stroll on the trail, you'll see a warm-up station where visitors can stretch before running. As the trail winds through the back of the park, you'll see a picnic pavilion to the right and baseball fields to the left.

Cross South Scenic Drive and walk toward another lake. Turn left at the path and continue walking around the lake. If it's summertime, you'll soon hear the sounds of children frolicking in the spray park. On the other side is a carousel, which, unlike the spray park, is open all year. A nearby snack bar offers a variety of cool treats, though hours vary.

Walk toward Downs and turn right before crossing the street. Walk past the soccer fields and cross over several parking lots until you reach the lot where you started.

## Point of Interest

**1** Lafreniere Park lafrenierepark.org, 3000 Downs Blvd., Metairie, 504-838-4389

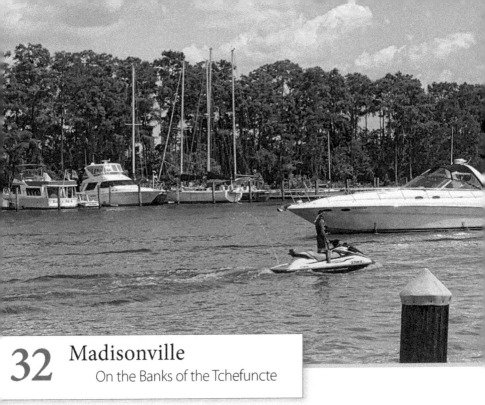

## 32 Madisonville
### On the Banks of the Tchefuncte

Above: The Tchefuncte River in Madisonville is a boat-lover's paradise.

DISTANCE: 1.4 miles
BOUNDARIES: Main St., Water St., St. Tammany St., Pine St., Jahncke St.
PARKING: Street parking, parking lot
PUBLIC TRANSIT: None

The town of Madisonville, about 30 miles north of New Orleans, is a boat lover's haven, the Tchefuncte River drawing residents and visitors alike to its inviting waters. On any given day, from Riverside Park, which lines the banks of the river, you'll see sailboats, yachts, skiffs, and any number of other floating vessels cruising this historic waterway.

The Tchefuncte (pronounced *chuh-funk-ta*) is a 70-mile river that winds through Washington, Tangipahoa, and St. Tammany Parishes, but it's the portion that flows through Madisonville in St. Tammany where so much of the fun takes place.

The merriment includes the annual Wooden Boat Festival, which attracts hundreds of handcrafted wooden boats from across the Gulf Coast. Presented by Lake Pontchartrain Basin Maritime Museum, the festival benefits educational programs along with the restoration of the Madisonville lighthouse.

The town's other premier event is Krewe of Tchefuncte Boat Parade, which takes place annually two weekends before Mardi Gras. Decorated boats start at nearby Salty's Marina, float south to the Maritime Museum, then head to the north side of the Madisonville Bridge before docking at the riverfront, where costumed riders toss beads and other throws to parade-goers.

Bear in mind you don't need a big event to enjoy Madisonville, a town of just over 800 people. There are any number of restaurants on Water Street, where you can grab a riverfront table and enjoy a plate of seafood while catching a glimpse of the passing boats. You can also sign up for a customized pontoon boat ride along the Tchefuncte. Check out louisiananorthshore.com for tour companies.

## Walk Description

Begin this walk at the ❶ Lake Pontchartrain Basin Maritime Museum, which aims to bring Louisiana's maritime history to life through interpretive programs, exhibits, children's programming, and events such as the annual Wooden Boat Festival. Among other things, the museum offers boat building, water safety, and aquatic robotic demonstrations. Exhibits include *Lighthouses of Louisiana* and *Civil War Submarine: The Pioneer.*

From the museum, walk five blocks to St. Louis Street. This is mostly a residential neighborhood that will take you past the Madisonville branch of the ❷ St. Tammany Parish Library to your right, just past Mabel Drive, and the Madisonville Ball Park to your left, just past Jahncke Street.

Turn right on St. Louis, walk one block to Water Street, and turn left. Water Street is where the action is in Madisonville. Stretching four blocks along the Tchefuncte River, it features numerous restaurants to your left and Riverside Park, a narrow greenspace that fronts the river, to your right.

In the first block of Water Street is the ❸ Water Street Bistro, a cozy and quaint eatery housed in a converted shotgun house. Chef Tony Monroe specializes in contemporary Louisiana cuisine, offering such dishes as sautéed crab cakes, pan-seared sea scallops, and Scotch smoked salmon.

Walk a block to St. Frances Street, where you'll see ❹ Madisonville Town Hall, home of the Madisonville city government. As of this writing, the city was studying a plan to convert the area into a quadrangle with a stage for performances, pavilions for farmers markets, and a boardwalk that would extend over the Tchefuncte River and include a gazebo.

Walk another block to the corner of Water and Mulberry Streets. At the corner is ⑤ Morton's Boiled Seafood and Bar, where the menu includes an array of shrimp, catfish, oyster, and softshell crab dishes. One of its signature cocktails is the Funky Tchefuncte, a concoction of Stoli orange with blue Pucker that, according to the menu, "arrives at the color of the river."

Cross Mulberry Street and continue on Water Street. Mulberry (LA 22) is a busy thoroughfare, and traffic often backs up when the bridge over the Tchefuncte is raised to let boats pass through. So be extra-cautious when you cross. At the corner is ⑥ Madisonville Riverside Bar, where you can play pool, watch a sporting event, or partake in daily happy hour from 4 to 7 p.m. Next door is ⑦ Water Street Wreaths, which sells handmade wreaths for practically every holiday and occasion and hosts wreath-making parties.

Continue on Water Street past ⑧ Abita Roasting Co., which has an inviting porch perfect for sipping a cup of freshly roasted coffee or any number of other coffee drinks. Feel free to take your coffee to one of the benches in Riverside Park, where you can get a closer view of the river as well as the riverside mansions on the other side.

Walk to the end of Water Street, about a half block down, and turn left on St. Tammany Street. As you make the turn, you'll notice two more restaurants. One is ⑨ The Anchor, which, in addition to a menu featuring fresh Louisiana seafood, has an outdoor game area, live music, and dockside boat parking. Just next door is ⑩ Tchefuncte's Restaurant, an upscale eatery with waterfront dining and a menu that includes an extensive selection of steak and seafood. The Anchor and Tchefuncte's are part of the same family.

Walk two blocks to Pine Street, turn left, and walk two more blocks to Mulberry Street, past ⑪ Madisonville Presbyterian Church, ⑫ Pad Thai restaurant, and ⑬ Kool Breeze Snowballs, the latter two of which face Mulberry. Cross Mulberry Street and continue on Pine three blocks past ⑭ Hopewell Baptist Church, several businesses, and ⑮ Madisonville Market, where, if it's a Sunday from 10 a.m. to 2 p.m., you'll have no choice but to make a stop. Presented by the Northshore Maker's Market Foundation, Madisonville Market, between St. Louis and Jahncke Streets, is a farmers market featuring more than 40 vendors selling ready-to-eat foods, baked goods, jams and jellies, sauces and seasonings, local honey, flowers, plants, eggs, cheese, fruit, and vegetables. Artisans selling original art, handmade jewelry, wooden creations, hand-dyed fabrics, and body care products are also on-site.

Turn left on Jahncke Street and walk one block to Main Street. Turn right on Main, and head back to the starting point two blocks down at Main and Mabel Drive. Although not included in this walk, consider a stop at Madisonville's ⑯ Fairview Riverside State Park, a 99-acre park that offers paddling, fishing, hiking, and overnight camping.

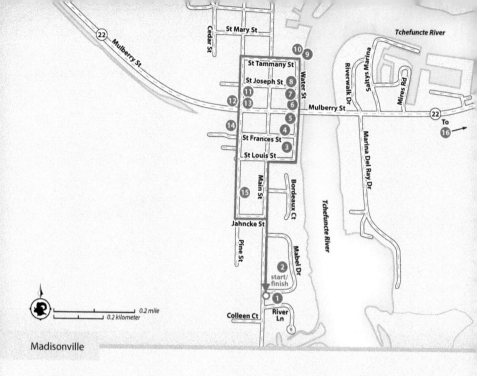

Madisonville

## Points of Interest

1. Lake Pontchartrain Basin Maritime Museum lpbmm.org, 133 Mabel Dr., Madisonville, 985-845-9200

2. St. Tammany Parish Library sttammanylibrary.org, 1123 Main St., Madisonville, 985-845-4819

3. Water Street Bistro 804 Water St., Madisonville, 985-845-3855

4. Madisonville Town Hall townofmadisonville.org, 403 St. Francis St., Madisonville, 985-845-7311

5. Morton's Boiled Seafood and Bar mortonsseafood.com, 702 Water Street, Madisonville, 985-845-4970

6. Madisonville Riverside Bar facebook.com/MadisonvilleRiversideBar, 708 Water St., Madisonville, 985-845-3731

7. Water Street Wreaths 700 Water St., Madisonville, 985-792-7979

8. Abita Roasting Co. abitaroasting.com, 504 Water St., Madisonville, 985-246-3340

9. The Anchor theanchorla.com, 407 St. Tammany St., Madisonville, 985-323-4800

10. Tchefuncte's Restaurant tchefunctes.com, 407 St. Tammany St., Madisonville, 985-323-4800

11 Madisonville Presbyterian Church  facebook.com/MadisonvillePresbyterianChurch, 705 Pine St., Madisonville, 985-845-8901

12 Pad Thai  302 LA 22 (Mulberry St.), Madisonville, 985-845-1888

13 Kool Breeze Snowballs  209 LA 22 (Mulberry St.), Madisonville, 985-845-9538

14 Hopewell Baptist Church  806 Pine St., Madisonville, 985-845-3317

15 Madisonville Market  madisonvillemarket.com, Pine St. between St. Louis and Jahncke Sts., Madisonville, 985-264-2328

16 Fairview Riverside State Park  lastateparks.com/parks-preserves/fairview-riverside-state-park, 119 Fairview Dr., Madisonville, 985-845-3318

*The homes of some Madisonville residents overlook the Tchefuncte River.*

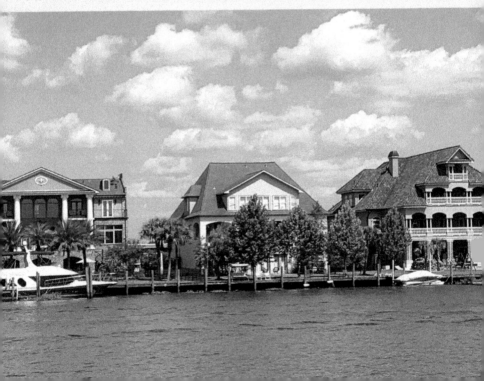

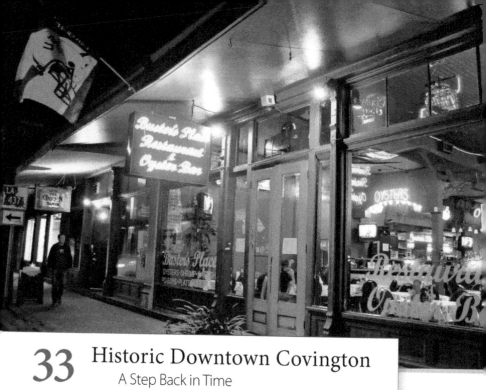

# 33  Historic Downtown Covington
## A Step Back in Time

*Above: Buster's Place Restaurant & Oyster Bar is one of the many dining destinations to consider on East Boston Street.    photo courtesy of the St. Tammany Parish Tourist Commission*

BOUNDARIES: E. Rutland St., Lee Lane, E. Lockwood St., N. Vermont St.
PARKING: Free on the street, but check signs for time limits
DISTANCE: 1.38 miles
PUBLIC TRANSIT: None

St. Tammany Parish, on the North Shore of Lake Pontchartrain, is home to a thriving collection of communities, from Abita Springs to Madisonville to Slidell. The city of Covington is among them, boasting such attractions as riverside parks, horse farms, and a historic downtown district.

Founded as the town of Wharton in 1813 but later renamed after Gen. Leonard Covington, a War of 1812 hero, the so-called Three Rivers community lies at the fork of the Bogue Falaya, Tchefuncte, and Abita Rivers. The downtown area thrived for decades but fell victim to the oil bust of

1986, forcing many businesses to shut down. In 1987, the city applied to and was accepted into the National Main Street Program, a downtown-revitalization initiative that started Covington's comeback in 1992.

The downtown district combines historic landmarks such as the Southern Hotel and H. J. Smith & Son General Store and Museum with modern and hip destinations such as Del Porte Ristorante, St. John's Coffeehouse, and the Green Room. Unique to the city is its grid layout, featuring squares-within-squares, or ox lots, that are accessible through alleyways and are now used for public parking.

The area also boasts a performing-arts center and several bed-and-breakfasts, all just steps away from the Bogue Falaya River and Bogue Falaya Park. Numerous art galleries also dot the streets, and every year, the Three River Arts Festival enhances the area's reputation as an arts and art lovers' Mecca.

## Walk Description

Begin on Lee Lane and East Gibson Street. Facing Lee Lane, turn left and walk two blocks to East Rutland Street. Lee Lane is a quaint two-block stretch of boutiques, galleries, and restaurants. These include ❶ Meribo, where happy hour features $7 pizzas; ❷ Ballin's, a high-end clothing store; ❸ Coffee Rani, one of the best salad spots in town; ❹ Mallie, another clothing boutique; and ❺ New Orleans Food and Spirits, known for its Cajun cooking.

Turn right on East Rutland and walk four blocks to North Vermont Street. On this part of the walk, you'll pass many turn-of-the-century cottages, some of which have been converted to businesses, such as ❻ On a Whim, which specializes in collectibles, antiques, and furniture, and the ❼ English Tea Room, which, in addition to breakfast and lunch, offers high tea all day.

At the intersection of East Rutland and North Columbia Street, to the left, is the Columbia Street Landing, which sits along the banks of the Bogue Falaya River. ❽ Bogue Falaya Park is just off North New Hampshire Street. The park is not included on this tour, but feel free to detour and then make your way back to East Rutland, where on your way to North Vermont Street you'll pass several bed-and-breakfasts, including ❾ Blue Willow and ❿ Camellia House.

At North Vermont Street, turn right and then right again onto East Boston Street, the district's main drag. At 428 E. Boston is the renovated ⑪ Southern Hotel, which opened in 1907 as a retreat for visitors who enjoyed the nearby piney woods and mineral springs. The hotel closed in the 1960s, and over the next several decades, the property housed a drugstore, government offices, and courthouses. After Hurricane Katrina, it served as the headquarters for the Red Cross and various federal agencies. Local developers bought the property in 2011 and set out to restore and reopen it as a luxury hotel. In addition to its 42 guest rooms, the hotel has a lush courtyard, a ballroom, an upscale bar, a fitness room, and spa services. Its restaurant, ⑫ Oxlot 9, boasts an award-winning chef, Jeffrey Hansell, who worked under Tory McPhail, chef of Commander's Palace. Other dining destinations on East Boston include ⑬ Del Porto Ristorante, ⑭ Vazquez Seafood & Po-Boy, and ⑮ Buster's Place Restaurant & Oyster Bar.

Walk two blocks to North Columbia Street, cross East Boston, and walk three blocks to East Lockwood Street. On North Columbia, you'll find ⑯ H. J. Smith and Sons General Store and Museum, a Covington institution since 1876. The store sells everything from hardware and army surplus to coonskin caps and rubber boots. Among the items on display at the museum are a hand-operated washing machine, a 1920s gas pump, and other memorabilia from the 1870s through the early part of the 20th century.

Just down the block at 320 N. Columbia is the home of the ⑰ St. Tammany Art Association, which was founded in 1958 by a small group of individuals dedicated to bringing the arts to west St. Tammany Parish. The association helps promote emerging and established artists, in addition to offering arts education and exhibitions. Every year, the group sponsors the Geaux Arts Ball, which raises money for its educational-outreach program.

Restaurants on North Columbia include ⑱ Pepe's, a fun spot to chill with a glass of wine or a margarita; the ⑲ Rock-N-Blues Café; and ⑳ Columbia Street Tap Room, which serves 30 beers on tap and 60 varieties of bottled beer.

Turn left at East Lockwood Street and walk one block to North New Hampshire Street. To your right is ㉑ Once in a While, a gift store with its own in-house coffee shop. Turn left on North New Hampshire and stop at the ㉒ Covington Trailhead, which marks the beginning of a 31-mile paved trail called the Tammany Trace. The trail connects Covington with the cities of Abita Springs, Mandeville, Lacombe, and Slidell. The site has a clock tower, an amphitheater, a museum and visitor center, and a small movie theater. You'll also see the world's tallest statue of President Ronald Reagan. On Wednesdays, the ㉓ Covington Farmers Market sets up shop here, selling locally grown fruits and vegetables, as well as locally produced eggs, milk, cheese, meat, poultry, and seafood. Musical performances and cooking demonstrations add to the festivities.

Continue two blocks on North New Hampshire back to East Boston Street, then turn left, and walk two blocks to North Florida Street. If you need a place to rest your feet and sip a drink, ㉔ Wharton's Green Room music club begins its happy hour at 2 p.m. For lattes and other coffee drinks, try ㉕ St. John's Coffeehouse. If you need a sugar fix, head to ㉖ Cupcake Concept, between North Columbia and North Florida Streets.

At North Florida, turn left and walk one block to East Gibson Street. Turn right and walk one block back to the starting point on Lee Lane.

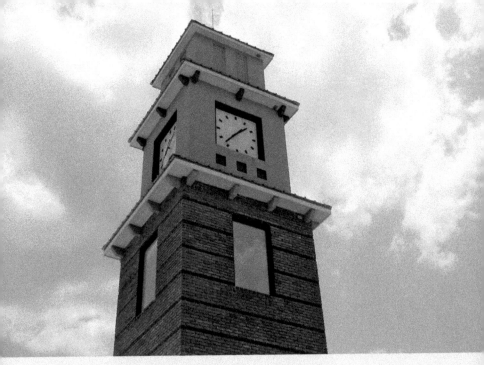

*The Covington Trailhead of the Tammany Trace features a bandstand, a visitor center, and this clock tower.*

## Points of Interest

1. Meribo  meribopizza.com, 326 Lee Lane, 985-302-5533
2. Ballin's  ballinsltd.com, 806 E. Boston St., 985-892-0025
3. Coffee Rani  coffeerani.com, 234 Lee Lane, 985-893-6158
4. Mallie  facebook.com/mallieboutique, 281 Lee Lane, 985-400-5220
5. New Orleans Food and Spirits  neworleansfoodandspirits.com, 208 Lee Lane, 985-875-0432
6. On a Whim  m4144.webnode.com, 826 E. Rutland St., 985-960-2117
7. English Tea Room  englishtearoom.com, 734 E. Rutland St., 985-898-3988
8. Bogue Falaya Park  213 Park Dr., 985-892-1873
9. Blue Willow Bed and Breakfast  bluewillowbandb.com, 505 E. Rutland St., 985-892-0011
10. Camellia House Bed and Breakfast  426 E. Rutland St., 985-264-4973
11. Southern Hotel  southernhotel.com, 428 E. Boston St., 844-866-1907
12. Oxlot 9  oxlot9.com, 428 E. Boston St., 985-400-5663

*(continued on next page)*

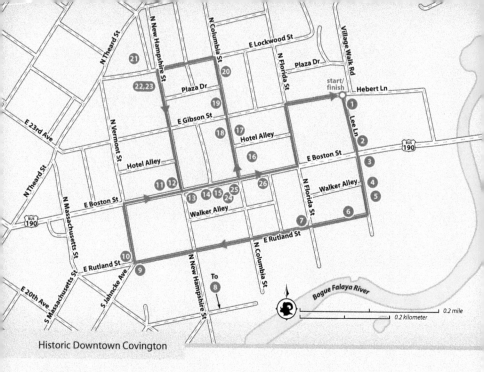

Historic Downtown Covington

*(continued from previous page)*

13. Del Porto Ristorante  delportoristorante.com, 501 E. Boston St., 985-875-1006

14. Vazquez Seafood & Po-Boy  vazquezpoboy.com, 515 E. Boston St., 985-893-9336

15. Buster's Place Restaurant & Oyster Bar  facebook.com/bustersplace, 519 E. Boston St., 985-809-3880

16. H. J. Smith and Sons General Store and Museum  308 N. Columbia St., 985-892-0460

17. St. Tammany Art Association  sttammany.art, 320 N. Columbia St., 985-892-8650

18. Pepe's  facebook.com/PepesCovington, 321 N. Columbia St., 985-400-5559

19. Rock-N-Blues Café  rocknbluescafe.com, 407 N. Columbia St., 985-892-9949

20. Columbia Street Tap Room  covingtontaproom.com, 434 N. Columbia St., 985-898-0899

21. Once in a While  greeneyedgoddess.com, 226 E. Lockwood St., 985-900-2227

22. Tammany Trace, Covington Trailhead  tammanytrace.org, 419 N. New Hampshire St., 985-867-9490

23. Covington Farmers Market  covingtonfarmersmarket.org, Covington Trailhead, 419 N. New Hampshire St., 985-966-1786

24. Wharton's Green Room  521 E. Boston St., 985-892-2225

25. St. John's Coffeehouse  stjohnscoffeehouse.com, 535 E. Boston St., 985-893-5553

26. Cupcake Concept  cupcakeconcept.com, 611 E. Boston St., 985-898-0400

# Appendix: Walks By Theme

## Art, Inside and Out

Audubon Park (Walk 13)
Contemporary Arts Center (Walk 1, Warehouse District)
Jazz Walk of Fame (Walk 26, Algiers Point)
Julia Street (Walk 1, Warehouse District)
Lafitte Greenway (Walk 18)
Louis Armstrong Park (Walk 21, Treme)
Magazine Street (Walk 11)
New Orleans Museum of Art (Walk 19, City Park)
North Columbia Street (Walk 33, Historic Downtown Covington)
Ogden Museum of Southern Art (Walk 1, Warehouse District)
Royal Street (Walk 4, French Quarter)
St. Claude Avenue (Walk 24)
Sydney and Walda Besthoff Sculpture Garden (Walk 19, City Park)
Woldenberg Riverfront Park (Walk 6, French Market/Riverfront)

## Dining, Shopping, and Entertainment

Bywater (Walk 23)
Esplanade Avenue (Walk 20, Faubourg St. John)
French Quarter (Walk 4, French Quarter; Walk 5, Back of the Quarter; Walk 6, French Market/Riverfront)
Frenchmen Street (Walk 22, Faubourg Marigny)
Freret Street (Walk 14)
Harrah's New Orleans (Walk 2, Canal Street; Walk 3, Poydras Street)
Harrison Avenue (Walk 29, Lakeview)
Lee Lane (Walk 33, Historic Downtown Covington)
Magazine Street (Walk 11)
Metairie Road (Walk 30, Old Metairie)
North Carrollton Avenue (Walk 17, Mid-City)
Oak Street (Walk 16, Carrollton)
Outlet Collection at Riverwalk (Walk 1, Warehouse District)
Riverbend (Walk 16, Carrollton)
St. Claude Avenue (Walk 24)
The Shops at Canal Place (Walk 2, Canal Street)
Shops at Jax Brewery (Walk 6, French Market/Riverfront)
Warehouse District (Walk 1)

## Family Fun

Audubon Aquarium of the Americas (Walk 6, French Market/Riverfront)
Audubon Park and Audubon Zoo (Walk 13)
City Park (Walk 19)

## Family Fun *(continued)*

**Crescent Park** (Walk 23, Bywater)
**Entergy IMAX Theatre** (Walk 6, French Market/Riverfront)
**French Market** (Walk 6, French Market/Riverfront)
**Jean Lafitte Barataria Preserve** (Walk 27)
**Lafreniere Park** (Walk 31)
**Louisiana Children's Museum** (Walk 19, City Park)

## Green Spaces

**Audubon Park** (Walk 13)
**Bogue Falaya Park** (Walk 33, Historic Downtown Covington)
**Chalmette Battlefield and National Cemetery** (Walk 25)
**City Park** (Walk 19)
**Coliseum Square** (Walk 7, Lower Garden District)
**Crescent Park** (Walk 23, Bywater)
**Jackson Square** (Walk 4, French Quarter)
**Jean Lafitte Barataria Preserve** (Walk 27)
**Lafayette Square** (Walk 1, Warehouse District)
**Lafitte Greenway** (Walk 18)
**Lafreniere Park** (Walk 31)
**Lakeshore Drive** (Walk 28, Lakefront)
**Louis Armstrong Park** (Walk 21, Treme)
**Washington Square** (Walk 22, Faubourg Marigny)
**Woldenberg Riverfront Park** (Walk 6, French Market/Riverfront)

## Hollywood South: Movie and TV Locations

*American Horror Story: Coven* (Walk 5, Back of the Quarter; Walk 12, St. Charles Avenue; Walk 14, Freret Street)
*Chef* (Walk 22, Faubourg Marigny)
*The Curious Case of Benjamin Button* (Walk 10, Garden District; Walk 22, Faubourg Marigny)
*Django Unchained* (Walk 10, Garden District)
*Double Jeopardy* (Walk 10, Garden District)
*The Expendables* (Walk 19, City Park)
*Interview with the Vampire* (Walk 5, Back of the Quarter; Walk 10, Garden District)
*NCIS: New Orleans* (Walk 1, Warehouse District; Walk 22, Faubourg Marigny)
*Now You See Me* (Walk 19, City Park)
*Pretty Baby* (Walk 12, St. Charles Avenue)
*Top Chef: New Orleans* (Walk 11, Magazine Street)
*Treme* (Walk 21)
*True Detective* (Walk 12, St. Charles Avenue)
*22 Jump Street* (Walk 15, University Area; Walk 19, City Park)

## Museums

Backstreet Cultural Museum (Walk 21, Treme)
The Cabildo (Walk 4, French Quarter)
Chalmette Battlefield Visitor Center (Walk 25)
Confederate Memorial Hall Museum (Walk 1, Warehouse District)
Contemporary Arts Center (Walk 1, Warehouse District)
H. J. Smith and Sons General Store and Museum (Walk 33, Historic Downtown Covington)
Historic New Orleans Collection (Walk 4, French Quarter)
Louisiana Children's Museum (Walk 19, City Park)
Lake Pontchartrain Basin Maritime Museum (Wak 32, Madisonville)
Museum of the Southern Jewish Experience (Walk 1, Warehouse District)
National World War II Museum (Walk 1, Warehouse District)
New Canal Lighthouse Museum and Education Center (Walk 28, Lakefront)
New Orleans African American Museum of Art, Culture and History (Walk 21, Treme)
New Orleans Jazz Museum (Walk 5, Back of the Quarter; Walk 22, Faubourg Marigny)
New Orleans Museum of Art (Walk 19, City Park)
Ogden Museum of Southern Art (Walk 1, Warehouse District)
Old Ursuline Convent Museum (Walk 5, Back of the Quarter)
Pharmacy Museum (Walk 4, French Quarter)
Pitot House (Walk 20, Faubourg St. John)
The Presbytère (Walk 4, French Quarter)
The Sazerac House (Walk 2, Canal Street)
Southern Food and Beverage Museum (Walk 8, Oretha Castle Haley Boulevard)
Treme's Petit Jazz Museum (Walk 21, Treme)

## Recovery and Rebirth

Bywater (Walk 23)
Freret Street (Walk 14)
Lakeview (Walk 29)
Lower Garden District (Walk 7)
Mid-City (Walk 17)
Oretha Castle Haley Boulevard (Walk 8)
St. Claude Avenue (Walk 24)

## Scary Stuff

Beauregard-Keyes House (Walk 5, Back of the Quarter)
Chalmette Battlefield and National Cemetery (Walk 25)
Cities of the Dead (Walk 17, Mid-City)
Lafayette Cemetery No. 1 (Walk 10, Garden District)
Lafitte's Blacksmith Shop (Walk 5, Back of the Quarter)
LaLaurie House (Walk 5, Back of the Quarter)

## Scary Stuff *(continued)*

**Madame John's Legacy** (Walk 5, Back of the Quarter)
**Marie Laveau's House of Voodoo** (Walk 5, Back of the Quarter)
**Mortuary Haunted House** (Walk 17, Mid-City)
**St. Louis Cemetery No. 1** (Walk 21, Treme)
**St. Louis Cemetery No. 3** (Walk 20, Faubourg St. John)

## Water, Water Everywhere

**Bayou St. John** (Walk 20, Faubourg St. John)
**Big Lake** (Walk 19, City Park)
**Lake Pontchartrain** (Walk 28, Lakefront)
**Louisiana wetlands** (Walk 27, Jean Lafitte Barataria Preserve)
**Mississippi River** (Walk 6, French Market/Riverfront; Walk 13, Audubon Park;
  Walk 23, Bywater; Walk 26, Algiers Point)
**Tchefuncte River** (Walk 32, Madisonville)

*St. Louis Cathedral, the highlight of Jackson Square, is flanked by the Cabildo and the Presbytère.*
*photo by Shutterstock/pisaphotography*

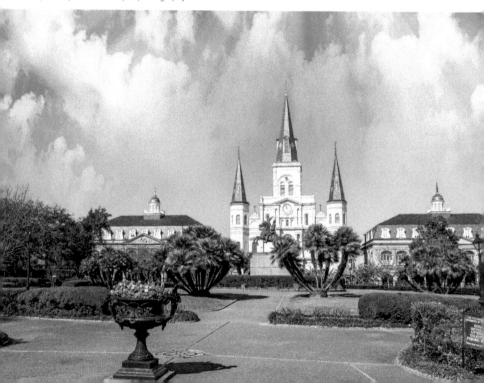

# Index

# About the Author

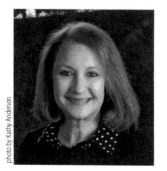

photo by Kathy Anderson

Barri Bronston is a lifelong New Orleanian who takes every opportunity to explore the city's neighborhoods, museums, parks, restaurants, and watering holes. She graduated with a bachelor's degree in journalism from the University of Missouri and spent most of her career as a staff writer at *The Times-Picayune*, where she covered parenting, education, and other topics. She is currently assistant director of public relations at Tulane University.